TOPICS IN DIETARY FIBER RESEARCH

TOPICS IN DIETARY FIBER RESEARCH

Edited by

Gene A. Spiller

Syntex Research
Palo Alto, California

With the assistance of

Ronald J. Amen

Syntex Research
Palo Alto, California

PLENUM PRESS · NEW YORK AND LONDON

Library of Congress Cataloging in Publication Data

Main entry under title:

Topics in dietary fiber research.

"A supplement to Fiber in human nutrition."
Includes bibliographies and index.
1. High-fiber diet. 2. Food—Fiber content. I. Spiller, Gene A. II. Fiber in human nutrition.
RM237.6.T66   612'.39   77-26883
ISBN-13: 978-1-4684-2483-6   e-ISBN-13: 978-1-4684-2481-2
DOI: 10.1007/978-1-4684-2481-2

© 1978 Plenum Press, New York
Softcover reprint of the hardcover 1st edition 1978
A Division of Plenum Publishing Corporation
227 West 17th Street, New York, N.Y. 10011

Preface

The study of plant fibers and their effect on human physiology has suddenly, after many years of comparative obscurity, been catapulted to the forefront of the scientific world. This new interest, first ignited by certain epidemiological reports, has been intensified by new research and by dramatization in the lay press. To counteract the dissemination of inaccurate information and to eliminate confusion, several authors have felt the need to make objective, unbiased reports available to the scientific community. The collection of papers in our own <u>Fiber in Human Nutrition</u> (Plenum Press, 1976) is one such effort. However, even as it was going to press, we realized that increased interest in specific areas of fiber research necessitated a more detailed and up-to-date look at certain topics. This book is directed to that purpose.

The first volume of <u>Fiber in Human Nutrition</u> was designed as a basic reference textbook covering the entire spectrum of plant fibers from chemical, analytical, physicochemical, physiological, medical and epidemiological points of view. The present volume, which enlarges on specific aspects of dietary fiber, is offered as a supplement to <u>Fiber in Human Nutrition</u>. Together, the two volumes should be a most valuable source of information for the student of the scientific intricacies of fiber.

An ongoing concern is that many of the substances dealt with in these and other "fiber" books are not, in the classical sense, of a fibrous nature at all. Efforts toward definitive nomenclature have produced a variety of terms: plantix, indigestible residue, partially digestible plant biopolymers, etc. Had this book been entitled "Selected Topics in Plantix Research," probably no one would have

known what it was about! Yet, undoubtedly, the term "fiber"
contains many linguistic weaknesses when applied to some of
the components of dietary fiber. Perhaps, with continuing
developments in the science of plant fibers in nutrition,
our next book may be published under a more accurate title.

                                        Gene A. Spiller
                                        Ronald J. Amen

Contents

CHAPTER 1

THE DETERGENT SYSTEM OF FIBER ANALYSIS

James B. Robertson

Animal Science Department, Cornell University

Ithaca, New York

I. INTRODUCTION

Hill (31) has postulated that the microflora of the gut produce carcinogens from, most probably, bile acids, and Visek (74) has suggested that ammonia, produced from microbial degradation of dietary protein in the lower gut, is a possible carcinogen. Both hypotheses are probably secondary to what seems to be the primary cause, a deficiency of dietary fiber which has been implicated in diverticular disease of the large bowel, carcinoma of the colon, ischemic heart disease, diabetes mellitus, and gallstone formation (9, 10, 14, 16, 27, 55, 58). Although by definition fiber is indigestible by the secretions of the gastrointestinal tract, there is sufficient evidence to show that the monogastric animal, in addition to the ruminant and nonruminant herbivore, has a microbial population (23) in the tract capable of utilizing plant structural carbohydrates as a source of energy (Table 1). However, no cellulolytic organisms have yet been isolated from human feces (35), although Bryant (8) has characterized strains of Rumunococcus and Bacteroides fragilis, many of which can ferment pentoses and possibly hemicelluloses.

II. SYSTEMS OF FIBER ANALYSIS

Thus, the assessment of foods for their fiber content and, perhaps even more so, for the composition of the fiber (i.e., hemicelluloses, cellulose, and lignin) and its poten-

TABLE 1. Fiber Digestibility in Various Species (percentages)

Animal	Substrate	Digestibility of				Source
		Cell wall	Hemicel-lulose	Cellulose	Crude Fiber	
Cow	Normal Diets					Arroyo-Aguilu and Evans (1)
	Range	32-71	44-84	3-79	--	
	Mean	55.8	68.0	51.6	--	
Horse	100% alfalfa	47.5	57.6	45.3	--	Hintz et al. (33)
	50% alfalfa, 50% grain	59.0	72.8	53.5	--	
	20% alfalfa, 80% grain	71.2	81.0	63.4	--	
Beaver	Normal diets	--	--	30.0	--	Hoover and Clarke (36)
Dog	Cereal-based diets	41.2	47.1	18.3	--	Visek and Robertson (74)
Meadow vole	100% alfalfa	33.9	39.1	33.6	--	Keys and Van Soest (40)
	75% brome	21.0	24.1	17.9	--	
	75% orchard grass	35.5	37.9	29.1	--	
Rat	Alfalfa	20.3	46.6	20.9	--	Keys et al. (41)
Sheep		44.9	46.5	50.1	--	
Swine		35.4	42.7	39.7	--	

TABLE 1. Fiber Digestibility in Various Species (percentages), Continued

Animal	Substrate	Cell wall	Hemicel-lulose	Cellulose	Crude fiber	Source
			Digestibility of			
Rat	Brome	5.4	10.7	0.5	--	Keys et al. (41)
Sheep		67.5	71.1	67.1	--	
Swine		43.0	46.7	38.5	--	
Rat	Orchard	8.4	6.4	1.5	--	Keys et al. (41)
Sheep	grass	69.7	76.3	67.4	--	
Swine		45.7	47.5	43.8	--	
Man	Wheat bran	30.1	--	--	--	Williams and Olmsted (79)
	Alfalfa leaf meal	8.8	--	--	--	
	Carrots	74.0	--	--	--	
	Corn germ meal	59.9	--	--	--	
	Cotton seed hulls	18.2	--	--	--	
	Sugar beet pulp	65.2	--	--	--	
	Peas	52.6	--	--	--	
	Cabbage	65.6	--	--	--	
	Agar-agar	59.0	59.0	--	--	
	Cellu flour®	10.5	--	10.5	--	

TABLE 1. Fiber Digestibility in Various Species (percentages), Continued

Animal	Substrate	Digestibility of				Source
		Cell wall	Hemicel-lulose	Cellulose	Crude fiber	
Man	All-Bran®	--	--	0.0	0.0	Hoppert and Clark (37)
	All-Bran®	--	--	6.0	5.0	
	Lettuce	--	--	29.0	0.0	
	Tomatoes	--	--	0.0	10.0	
	Cabbage	--	--	42.0	14.0	
	Celery	--	--	29.0	17.0	
	Oranges	--	--	24.0	28.0	
	Apples	--	--	57.0	71.0	
Man	Mixed diet					
	Range	31-72	54-80	54-85	--	Hummel et al. (38)
	Mean	48.1	66.6	70.9	--	
Man	Ground wheat	--	--	--	7.0	Crampton et al. (12)
Rat		--	--	--	10.0	
Guinea pig		--	--	--	36.0	
Sheep		--	--	--	-4.0	
Swine		--	--	--	15.0	
Man	Cracked wheat porridge	--	--	--	28.0	Crampton et al. (12)

TABLE 1. Fiber Digestibility in Various Species (percentages), Continued

Animal	Substrate	Digestibility of				Source
		Cell wall	Hemicel-lulose	Cellulose	Crude fiber	
Man	Shredded Wheat®	—	—	—	-7.0	Crampton et al. (12)
Rat		—	—	—	11.0	
Guinea pig		—	—	—	51.0	
Sheep		—	—	—	-17.0	
Swine		—	—	—	-23.0	
Man	No fruit or vege-tables except potato	—	94-98	15-55	—	Southgate and Durnin (54)
	Fruit, vegetables and whole wheat bread	—	72-85	15-44	—	
	Fruit, vegetables and whole wheat bread, high level	—	83.0	22.0	—	
Man	Corn, soybean, wheat bran, citrus fruit, purified cellulose	55.7-60.6	67.4-71.4	28.6-35.0	—	Raymond et al. (48)
Man	All-Bran®	57.0	68.0	51.0	—	Wrick (80)

tial digestibility is necessary if the role of fiber in the
diet is to be understood. One system of fiber analysis is
based on the use of detergents.

The apparatus and reagents used in the detergent
system of fiber analysis have been described by Goering
and Van Soest (25). The system has been based on the work
of Van Soest and his colleagues (62, 63, 64, 71, 72, 73).
It was developed primarily for evaluating ruminant diets
(65) but has found application in studying the diets of
other herbivores and nonruminants (17, 18, 19, 20, 33, 34,
36, 40, 41, 75).

All of the recent systems of fiber analysis (3, 6, 7,
22, 30, 51, 52, 53, 65) have been developed to replace the
Weende system of feed analysis, which consists of a nitrogen
determination, an ether extract, a total ash, and a crude-
fiber measurement (2). The difference between 100 and the
sum of N x 6.25, ether extract, ash, and crude fiber is
called the nitrogen-free extract and assumed to be soluble
carbohydrates.

The origin of the sequential extraction with solvent,
dilute aqueous acid, and dilute alkali in the crude fiber
determination is uncertain (59). Einhof, to whom the sequential extraction has been attributed, used only extensive
maceration of the plant tissue and extraction with cold and
hot water. By the time of Henneberg, it seems to have been
in common use. The crude-fiber method as an estimate of the
fiber in foods has many defects (68, 69). About 80% of the
pentosans, 50 to 90% of the lignin, and 20 to 50% of the
cellulose are removed by the acid and alkali extraction.
This has resulted in reports of some digestibility studies
in which the digestibility of the crude fiber was equal to
or greater than that of the nitrogen-free extract (Figure 1
and 2 and Table 2).

III. THE DETERGENT SYSTEMS

Because of the failure of the crude-fiber procedure to
recover the hemicelluloses, cellulose, and lignin of plant
tissue, other approaches have been taken. Reports had shown
that anionic detergents facilitate the solution of protein
in slightly alkaline solutions (5, 21, 78), and quaternary

TABLE 2.   Relative Digestibility of Crude Fiber
and NFE in Ruminants

Feed	Number of digestion trials	% of cases where digestibility of CF $\geq$ NFE
Dry feed	110[1]	30[1]
Succulent feed	61[1]	20[1]
Silage	25[1]	28[1]
Concentrates	88[1]	10[1]
Tropical forage	268[2]	66[2]

[1]Crampton and Maynard (13).

[2]Butterworth (11).

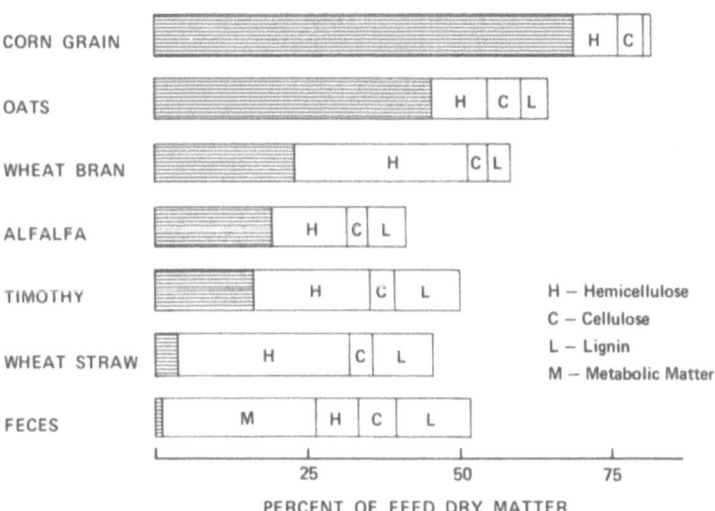

Figure 1.   The amount and composition of the NFE in some con-
centrates, forages, and feces.   Shaded bar indicates organic
acids and soluble carbohydrates.   Feces contain a large portion of metabolic matter, which represents the difference between true and apparent digestibility.   Based on data of Van
Soest, unpublished.

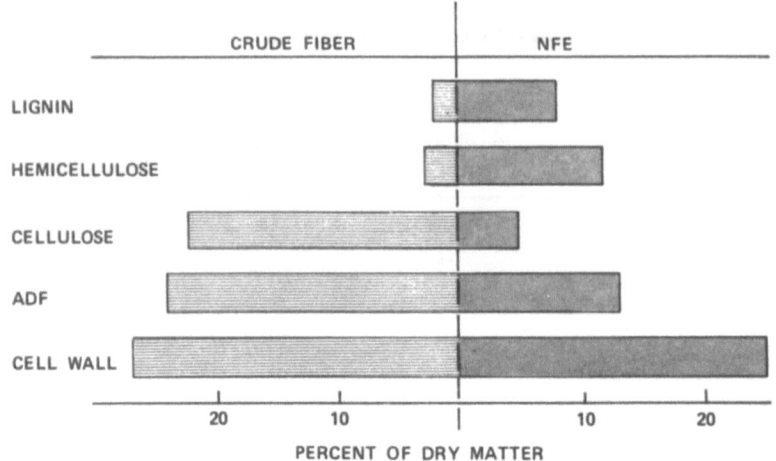

Figure 2. The relative amount and distribution of lignin, hemicellulose, cellulose, acid detergent fiber (ADF) and cell wall between crude fiber and NFE for an average alfalfa hay which contained 28% crude fiber and 41% NFE. Based on data of Van Soest, unpublished.

ammonium compounds (5, 39) dissolve polysaccharides, proteins, and nucleic acids. Van Soest (62) tested various anionic, cationic, and nonionic detergents in buffer solutions of various pH and measured the nitrogen, hemicelluloses, cellulose, and lignin in the residue of plant tissue treated with these solutions (Figure 3). A solution of sodium lauryl sulfate buffered at pH 7 with EDTA-borate recovers the hemicelluloses, cellulose, and lignin in the residue and solubilizes over 75% of the nitrogen. Cetyl trimethylammonium bromide in INH_2SO_4 (pH < 1) recovers the cellulose and lignin in the residue while removing more than 95% of both the hemicelluloses and nitrogen. Lignin does contain some nitrogen ($\sim$2%). The acid-detergent residue, with its low nitrogen content, is a suitable start for the Klason (72%-H_2SO_4) lignin procedure. An alternative lignin procedure is that which utilizes permanganate (72). Potassium permanganate oxidizes lignin and other aromatic compounds in plant tissue but does not attack cellulose.

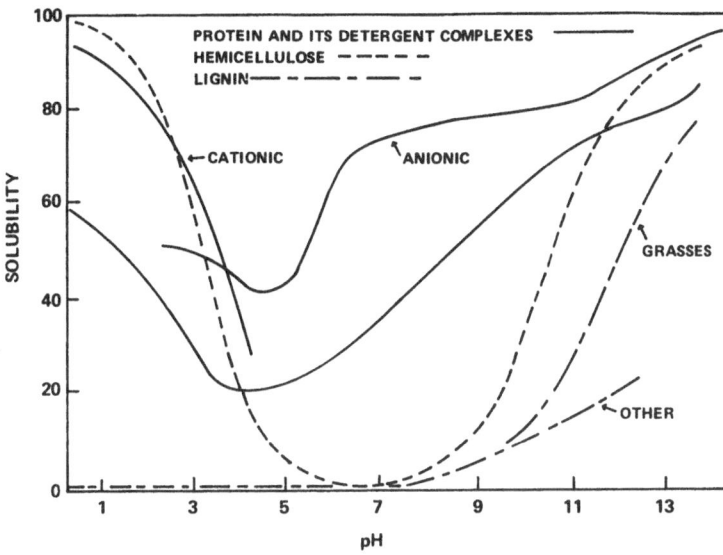

Figure 3. The relative solubility of forage hemicellulose, lignin, protein, and protein-detergent complexes in boiling aqueous medium at different pH. Reproduced with permission from Van Soest (67).

IV. NUTRITIONAL IMPLICATIONS OF THE DETERGENT SYSTEMS

Although the neutral detergent (ND) and acid detergent (AD) residues overcome the deficiencies of the crude fiber procedure in that they recover the structural components of the plant tissue, they are of little value unless they have nutritional implications. The validity of the detergent system of partitioning forage dry matter into fractions of similar nutritional availability has been tested by the method of Lucas, Smart, Cipollini, and Gross (43). In the Lucas test, the digestible amount of the component to be tested is regressed upon the percentage of the component in the forage dry matter. The regression constant is an estimate of the average true digestibility of the component. Height of the correlation and the standard deviation of the regression are estimates of the uniform nutritional availability of the component.

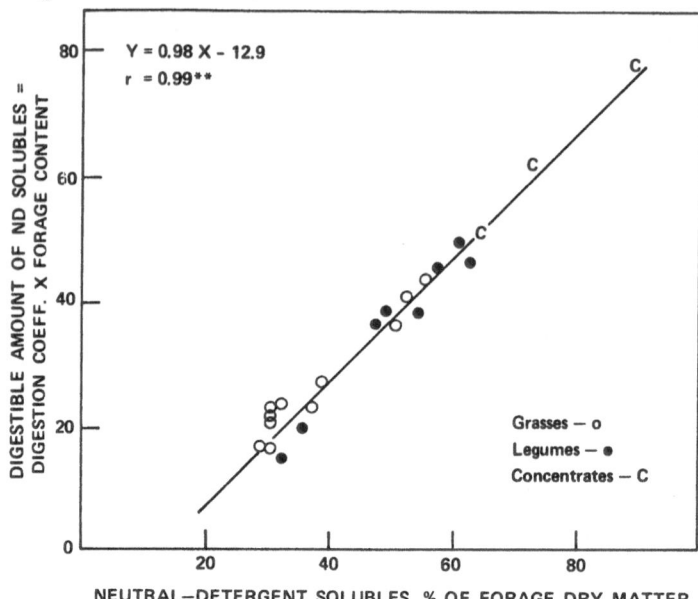

Figure 4. Relationship between the digestible amount of
cellular contents and total amount in the dry matter,
measured as dry matter soluble in neutral detergent. Reproduced with permission from Van Soest (67).

        The application of the Lucas test to a group of forages
fed to ruminants is illustrated in Figures 4, 5, and 6. In
Table 3 are typical regression equations obtained when the
test is made. Cellular contents (100-ND residue) and
N x 6.25 show a high degree of nutritional uniformity and
have true digestibilities approaching 100%. Lignin is a
component that shows nonnutritional uniformity. The cell
wall (NDR), hemicelluloses, and cellulose are nonuniform
nutritional components by the Lucas test.

        In part, the nutritional nonuniformity of cell wall,
hemicelluloses, and cellulose is due to their heterogeneous
chemical composition. Only the cellulose of cotton is a
homogeneous β-glucan. However, most of the nonuniformity can
be explained by the lignin content of the tissue (Table 4,
Figure 7). Lignin is chemically linked to the structural
polysaccharides and depresses their digestibility (28).

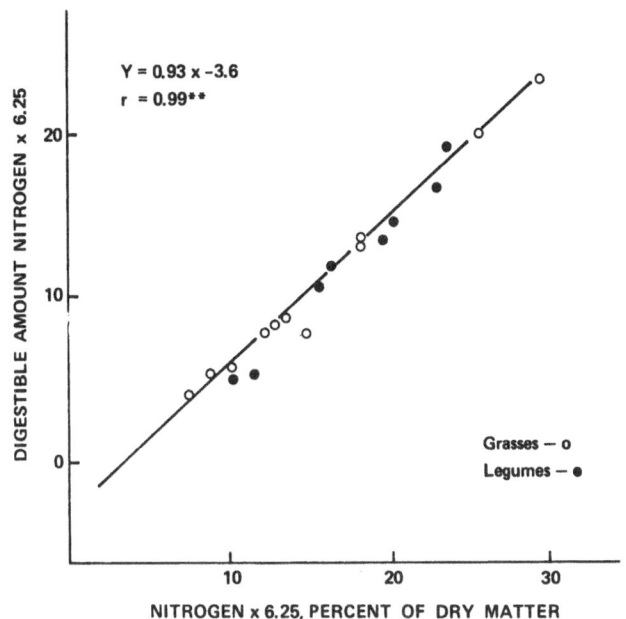

Figure 5. Relationship between digestible amount of nitrogen and the total amount in the dry matter. Based on data of Van Soest (54).

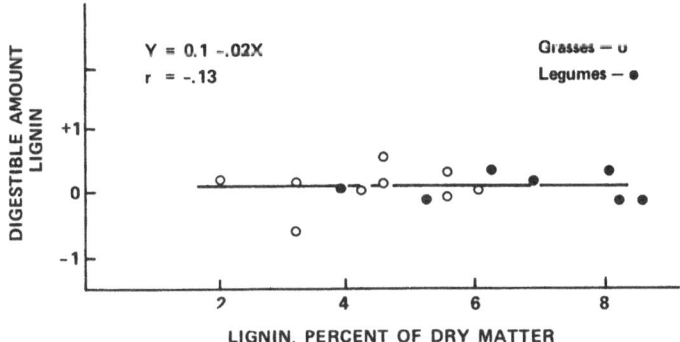

Figure 6. Relationship between the digestible amount of lignin and total amount in the dry matter. Based on data of Van Soest (54).

TABLE 3. Regressions of Apparent Digestible Amount on Contents of Various Fractions in Forages Fed to Ruminants[1]

Fraction	Mean apparent digestibility (%)	True digestibility[1] (b)	S_b	Endogenous excretion[2] (-a)	S_a
Soluble					
Cellular contents	66	98	2.5	12.9	2.1
Sugars	100	100	0.4	0.2	0.2
N x 6.25	68	93	3.1	3.6	0.8
Ether extract	67	86	6.6	1.1	0.4
Fibrous fractions					
Cell wall	59	62	14.1	1.3	7.4
Hemicellulose	66	79	6.7	-2.3	2.3
Cellulose	63	50	13.5	-3.9	3.8
Lignin	1	-2	3.7	-0.1	0.3
Other fractions					
Crude fiber	47	36	7.2	-7.1	2.6
NFE	72	61	8.9	-4.1	3.8
ADF	55	30	12.6	8.6	4.3

Source: Based on data of Lucas and Smart (43); Van Soest (66).

[1] Slope of regression of digestible amount on content x 100.

[2] Intercept of regression at zero content.

TABLE 4. Correlations of Digestible Amount with Forage Content, Estimates of Average True Digestibility, and Correlations of Apparent Digestibility with Indices of Lignification for Different Forage Fractions

Fraction	Correlation of digestible amount with content	Estimated true digestibility(%)[1]	Correlation of Apparent Digestibility with		
			Lignin/cell wall	Lignin/ADF[2]	Log lignin/ADF[2]
N x 6.25	0.99[3]	93 ± 3.1	-.14	-.16	-.21
Cellular contents	0.99[3]	98 ± 2.5	-.14	-.15	-.21
Cellulose	0.67[3]	50 ± 13.5	-.83[3]	-.91[3]	-.93[3]
Hemicellulose	0.94[3]	79 ± 6.7	-.85[3]	-.86[3]	-.90[3]
Acid-detergent fiber (ADF)	0.50[4]	30 ± 12.6	-.86[3]	-.93[3]	-.95[3]
Cell wall	0.73[3]	62 ± 14.1	-.90[3]	-.95[3]	-.98[3]

Source: From Van Soest and Moore (7C).

[1] Slope of the regression of digestible amount on forage content.

[2] Acid-detergent fiber.

[3] $P < .01$.

[4] $P < .05$.

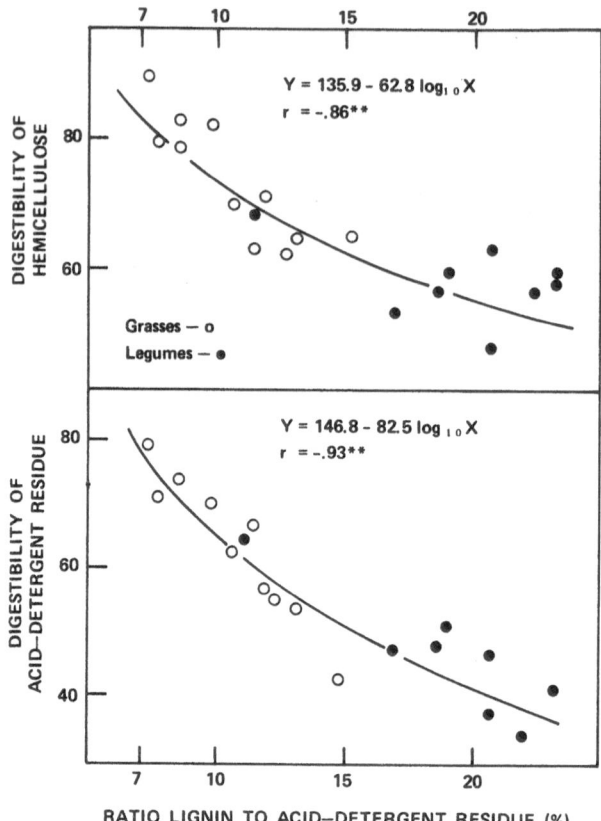

Figure 7. Curvilinear relationship between digestibility
of hemicellulose and acid-detergent fiber and the lignin
concentration in the acid-detergent fiber. Based on data
of Van Soest and Moore (58).

Using the logarithm of the ratio of lignin content to ADR
content, an estimate of the digestibility of the cell wall
by ruminants can be made (25).

     Thus, the detergent system of fractionating the forage
dry matter made it possible to classify the forage fractions
according to nutritive characteristics and estimate their
availability (digestibility) in ruminants (Table 5). The

TABLE 5. Basic Scheme of Forage Analysis Using Detergents

Fraction	Nutritional availability	Reagent	Treatment	Yield
Cell contents	Almost completely digestible		Calculate as 100 − NDR	Lipids, sugars, organic acids, starch, soluble protein, nucleic acids, pectin
Neutral-detergent residue (NDR)	Partially available depending on degree of lignification	Na lauryl sulfate, EDTA Borate pH 7.0	Boil 1 hr	Plant cell wall less pectins
Acid-detergent residue (ADR)	Partially available depending on degree of lignification	Cetyl tri-methyl-ammo-nium bromide in 1 N H_2SO_4	Boil 1 hr	Lignocellulose + insoluble minerals
Lignin	Unavailable	72%-H_2SO_4	3 hr at 20^oC	Crude lignin
Lignin	Unavailable	$KMnO_4$ pH 3.0	1-1/2 hr at 20°C	Lignin as loss in wt by oxidation
Cellulose	Partially available depending on degree of lignification	None	Ash residue from lignin step	Loss in wt
Cutin	Unavailable	72%-H_2SO_4	Treat cellu-lose 3 hr at 20°C	Residue is cutin
Silica (SiO_2)	Unavailable	Conc HBr (40%)	Treat ash drop-wise 1 hr at 20^oC	Residue is SiO_2
Hemicellulose	Partially available depending on degree of lignification	None	Calculate as NDR − ADR	--

Source: Spiller and Amen (55).

estimation of availability of the structural carbohydrates
to nonruminants must await the accumulation of sufficient
digestibility data to derive the necessary equations.

V.   IN-VITRO CELL-WALL DIGESTION

Although the structural carbohydrates are not digested
by gastrointestinal secretions, they do form a substrate for
the bacteria in the tract. Thus, in addition to partioning
the fiber (cell wall) into hemicelluloses, cellulose, and
lignin, the digestibility of the cell wall should be considered when evaluating dietary fiber. The digestion of
forage dry matter by rumen bacteria in vitro is a well-
developed procedure and shows a high correlation to in-vivo
values (57, 73). Waldo, Smith, and Cox (77) have suggested
that cellulose in the forage dry matter can be partioned
into an indigestible fraction and a potentially digestible
fraction. The degree of digestion of the potentially digestible fraction will depend on the rate of passage of that
fraction through the rumen. Waldo (76) has presented evidence
that although 90% of the cellulose digestion occurred in the
rumen, only 66 to 69% of the hemicellulose digestion occurred
there, the remainder occurring in the lower tract. Hintz,
Hogue, Walker, Lowe, and Schryver (33) showed that in ponies,
47% of the cell-wall digestion occurred in the colon.

Mertens (47) has developed models for cell-wall digestion in vitro. When cell wall was digested for various
periods of time and the residue remaining corrected for the
indigestible residue, it was found that the rate of digestion of the digestible cell wall followed the first order
kinetics (Figure 8).

From Figure 8 it can be seen that the length of time
to which cell wall is subjected to fermentation in vitro
will control the amount of undigested residue and also the
availability of energy from the fiber. This can be considered
in part equivalent to the effect of rate of passage or transit
time. A short transit time will result in a high fiber residue
whereas a long transit time will give maximum utilization of
fiber energy. Indirect evidence that this occurs in vivo has
been obtained through the study of the digestibility depres-
sion phenomenon in ruminants (49) or by the studies on stool
weight and transit time in humans (9). An alternative to

in-vitro rumen could be the development of techniques using aerobic cellulases from fungi (45, 69).

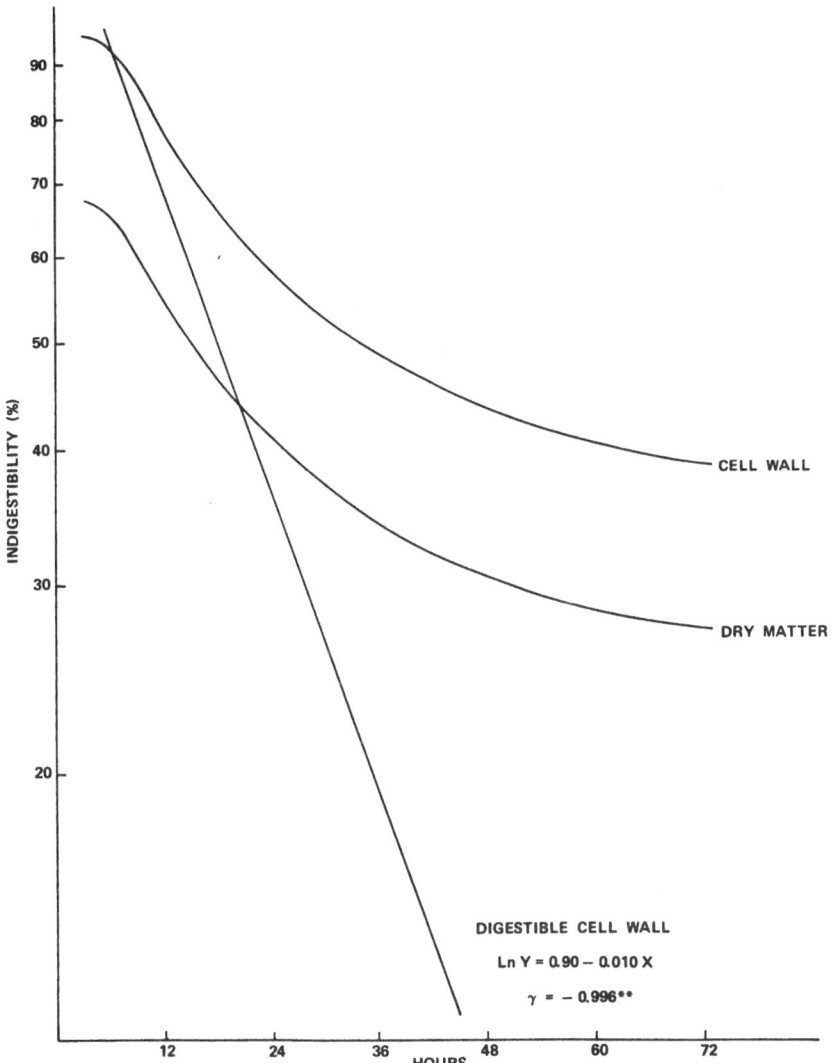

Figure 8. The in-vitro rumen indigestibility of dry matter, cell wall, and digestible cell wall (cell wall corrected for indigestible residue) of a grass.

Thus, the detergent system can fractionate food dry matter into dietary fiber (cell wall) and estimate the digestibility of that fiber by ruminants. By utilizing the in-vitro technique for measuring rate of cell-wall digestion, it should be possible to estimate the undigested fiber in monogastric diets.

VI. PROCEDURES IN THE DETERGENT SYSTEM OF FIBER ANALYSIS

The apparatus, reagents, and procedures have been described by Goering and Van Soest (25). Since that publication slight modifications have been made by Van Soest, and some parts of the procedures need redefining. The standard system as described in Agricultural Handbook No. 379 is capable of adaptation to the equipment and needs of the user, and this capability is one of the prime advantages of the detergent method of fiber analysis. Some typical detergent fiber analyses are given in Table 6.

The apparatus remains basically the same: a reflux unit, filtering manifold, and hot water supply. The hot water system described in the handbook requires that the water heating unit, preferably a 3-liter, 3-neck flask, be modified by a glassblower. It is not commercially available. Two alternatives are the hot water system described by the AOAC (2) for the crude-fiber procedure and an electric water heater such as that used in bomb calorimetry. The rubber adapters used in the original filtering manifold are apparently no longer available. Automobile radiator hose of suitable diameter may be substituted or "O" rings made from an old inner tube from a car. Stainless steel tubing might be used instead of polyethylene in the manifold. In the traps (4-liter filtering flasks) between the manifold and the vacuum source, an antifoaming agent is highly advantageous. Normal butyl alcohol or one of the silicone-based antifoamants may be used. Water-operated aspirators do not usually have the vacuum capacity to handle more than one or two filtrations simultaneously.

In addition to a reflux unit, hot water supply, and filtering manifold, miscellaneous glassware and other equipment are needed: beakers, Gooch crucibles, macroanalytical balance, oven, and furnace.

The Gooch crucibles should be 50 ml, high form with a fritted glass plate of coarse porosity (40 μ maximum pore size) and should be engraved with permanent identification numbers. These crucibles will melt or become misshapen if they are subjected to temperatures much above 500°C. Thus, the muffle furnace used for ashing should have precise temperature control for best results. The crucibles should not be removed from the furnace until the temperature has dropped below 250°C, and when they are removed, they should be placed on an asbestos sheet rather than directly on the metal surface of a pan. Eventually, the sinter glass plate of the crucible will become clogged with mineral matter and may be cleaned with strong, hot alkali.

A single-pan automatic balance sensitive to 0.1 mg should be used, preferably with digital rather than vernier readout. Since the crucibles are weighed at 100°C, the balance is subjected to heating and cooling and thus will not have a steady zero reading. Because of the construction of most balances, heating causes the balance to go negative. Thus, a positive tare must be put on the balance initially. Using the zero adjustment, put a positive optical tare of 8 to 10 mg on the balance. Remove crucible from the oven, place on pan, and record the weight when the minimum weight is obtained (about 20 to 30 sec after the crucible is placed on the pan). Remove crucible. Now record the optical tare on the balance. Weigh the next crucible, record optical tare, etc. For example:

	Grams
Initial optical tare	.0100
Crucible #1	37.2468
New tare	.0095
Crucible #2	34.4375
New tare	.0090
Crucible #3	36.1433
New tare	.0080

Grams

True weight of crucible #1 = 37.2468 − 0.0095 = 37.2373
True weight of crucible #2 = 34.4375 − 0.0090 = 34.4285
True weight of crucible #3 = 36.1433 − 0.0080 = 36.1353

TABLE 6. Fiber Composition of Some Foodstuffs (percentages)

Foodstuff	Dry matter	Cell wall	Lignin (KMnO$_4$)	In Dry Matter				
				Cellulose	Hemicelluloses	Crude fiber	Crude protein	Fiber-bound protein
Bread, white, enriched	64.2	2.4[1]	0.3	0.5	1.6	1.7	15.1	0.2
Bread, whole wheat	64.4	10.6[1]	1.6	2.3	6.7	5.1	18.6	0.8
Bran'nola® (Arnold)	64.23	6.67[1]	.68	1.69	4.30	-	17.04	-
Less® (J.J. Nissen)	55.71	16.80[1]	1.11	12.70	2.99	-	17.07	-
Fresh Horizons® White (I.T.T.)	54.21	18.44[1]	.78	15.58	2.08	-	17.20	-
All-Bran®	97.3	33.9[1]	2.7	6.8	24.4	9.2	11.6	0.5
Cornflakes	96.3	4.4[1]	1.5	2.0	0.9	1.4	7.9	2.8
Cheerios®	94.0	6.5[1]	1.8	1.4	3.3	2.7	17.0	1.6
Porridge oats	91.1	6.9[1]	1.1	1.0	4.8	2.0	12.9	0.3

Source: American Association of Cereal Chemists Conference, New Orleans, October 1976.
Note: The slight differences between the cell wall values and the sum of lignin, cellulose, and hemicellulose values may be a result of pectin and cutin contamination.
[1] Analyzed by the amylase modification of the neutral detergent fiber method (Van Soest and Robertson, 1976).

TABLE 6. Fiber Composition of Some Foodstuffs (percentages), Continued

Foodstuff	Dry matter	Cell wall	Lignin ($KMnO_4$)	Cellulose	Hemicelluloses	Crude fiber	Crude protein	Fiber-bound protein
Cauliflower	6.2	16.0	1.5	10.8	4.1	10.3	24.7	—
Celery	5.0	14.4	2.0	12.1	0.3	13.3	14.4	—
Collard greens	9.6	18.6	3.1	12.1	3.2	11.1	27.8	—
Corn, kernel, sweet	20.4	7.9[1]	1.9	2.6	3.4	2.2	13.8	—
Cucumber, peeled	3.2	12.7	1.7	9.1	2.0	13.4	15.3	—
Cucumber, skin	8.5	35.5	5.7	19.5	0.4	34.1	17.7	—
Eggplant, peeled	6.9	21.8	3.4	13.8	4.6	18.6	14.5	—
Kale	8.4	16.5	2.3	12.3	2.0	11.8	27.7	—
Lettuce, romaine	4.9	17.3	2.8	13.3	1.2	12.4	24.6	—
Mustard greens	7.6	21.7	3.1	14.4	4.1	13.5	31.2	—
Okra	7.5	14.1	1.6	9.2	3.3	9.3	20.6	—
Onions	6.6	7.6	0.6	6.2	0.9	6.1	9.2	—
Oranges, peeled	13.6	3.7[1]	1.8	1.7	0.2	2.7	7.0	—
Peas, black-eyed	35.0	9.0[1]	1.8	6.3	0.9	5.6	27.0	—
Peas, green, sweet	20.7	13.3	0.5	10.0	2.8	8.1	30.9	—
Pepper, seedless	9.9	17.2[1]	2.2	12.3	2.7	14.5	14.8	—
Potatoes, peeled	22.2	2.5	0.4	1.6	0.5	0.5	9.5	—

Source: American Association of Cereal Chemists Conference, New Orleans, October 1976.
Note: The slight differences between the cell wall values and the sum of lignin, cellulose, and hemicellulose values may be a result of pectin and cutin contamination.
[1] Analyzed by the amylase modification of the neutral detergent fiber method (Van Soest and Robertson, 1976).

TABLE 6. Fiber Composition of Some Foodstuffs (percentages), Continued

Foodstuff	Dry matter	Cell wall	Lignin (KMnO₄)	In Dry Matter				
				Cellu-lose	Hemi-cellu-loses	Crude fiber	Crude protein	Fiber-bound protein
Grape-Nuts®	94.9	8.2[1]	1.0	1.7	5.5	2.2	12.9	1.0
Puffed Wheat®	94.3	7.6[1]	2.3	2.2	3.1	3.5	17.2	2.2
Shredded Wheat®	93.5	13.4[1]	2.7	3.4	7.3	3.6	11.2	1.7
Wheat Chex®	96.4	9.6[1]	4.4	2.8	2.4	3.5	11.8	3.7
Wheaties®	95.3	11.1[1]	2.5	2.7	5.9	3.0	9.8	2.7
Heartland®	97.4	7.4[1]	1.2	0.9	5.3	6.0	13.5	0.5
Apples	11.7	7.6	0.1	4.7	2.9	3.7	1.3	—
Artichoke hearts	12.1	12.5	1.5	8.1	3.1	8.1	20.4	—
Asparagus	8.5	12.6	1.1	9.1	2.4	9.5	36.1	—
Beans, green, cut	7.7	17.6[1]	3.1	11.2	3.3	10.9	18.1	—
Beans, lima, baby	33.2	11.9[1]	0.8	7.4	3.7	6.1	19.3	—
Beans, wax, cut	8.5	18.7[1]	2.1	14.3	2.3	12.6	18.9	—
Beet root	12.5	11.8	0.1	5.3	6.5	4.7	10.9	—
Broccoli	7.3	18.4	2.7	-13.6	2.0	13.8	33.6	—
Brussels sprouts	10.2	21.9	1.8	13.0	7.4	12.2	23.9	—
Cabbage	7.8	14.2	0.7	9.8	3.7	8.4	12.5	—
Carrots	10.4	9.2	1.4	6.6	1.2	5.7	6.8	—

Source: American Association of Cereal Chemists Conference, New Orleans, October 1976.
Note: The slight differences between the cell wall values and the sum of lignin, cellu-lose, and hemicellulose values may be a result of pectin and cutin contamination.
[1] Analyzed by the amylase modification of the neutral detergent fiber method (Van Soest and Robertson, 1976).

TABLE 6. Fiber Composition of Some Foodstuffs (percentages), Continued

Foodstuff	Dry matter	Cell wall	Lignin (KMnO$_4$)	In Dry Matter				
				Cellu-lose	Hemi-cellu-loses	Crude fiber	Crude protein	Fiber-bound protein
Potatoes, skin	18.2	12.9[1]	6.5	5.0	1.4	9.8	16.1	—
Radishes	11.9	14.3	1.2	7.6	5.5	11.4	17.1	—
Rutabaga, peeled	10.0	10.2	1.6	6.8	1.8	7.4	13.4	—
Spinach	7.6	17.6	2.2	11.4	3.8	11.1	27.5	—
Squash, summer	5.0	11.4[1]	1.7	8.1	1.6	7.5	20.6	—
Squash, zucchini	4.6	12.5[1]	1.6	8.8	2.1	9.0	18.9	—
Squash, cooked	9.8	13.6[1]	0.7	10.5	2.4	7.5	20.6	—
Turnip greens	6.6	19.4	2.8	15.2	1.4	13.8	34.9	—
Bran, bakers	91.6	37.2[1]	2.9	7.5	26.8	9.9	21.4	—
Bran, cereal	90.4	45.4[1]	4.5	10.8	30.3	11.7	19.7	—

Source: American Association of Cereal Chemists Conference, New Orleans, October 1976.
Note: The slight differences between the cell wall values and the sum of lignin, cellulose, and hemicellulose values may be a result of pectin and cutin contamination.
[1] Analyzed by the amylase modification of the neutral detergent fiber method (Van Soest and Robertson, 1976).

A sequence of weighing will result such that one
crucible is weighed/min. To heat up the balance, two blank
crucibles should be weighed first. After weighing 10 crucibles, the optical tare will stabilize. It is advisable to
weigh crucibles in a set order for best accuracy. If there
are wide fluctuations in room temperature and humidity,
standardizing crucibles should be included in the weighing
sequence, since room conditions will affect the balance.

The reagents used are essentially similar to those
previously described (25) but for convenience are repeated
below.

A.   Reagents

Neutral Detergent Solution. The following will make
about 18 l neutral detergent solution.

Distilled water	18.0 l
Sodium lauryl sulfate, laboratory grade	540.0 g
Ethylene diamine tetra-acetic acid, A.C.S.	263.0 g
Sodium hydroxide, A.R.	72.0 g
Sodium borate dicahydrate, A.R.	122.6 g
Disodium hydrogen phosphate, anhydrous, A.R.	82.1 g
Ethylene glycol monoethyl ether, purified grade	180.0 ml

The H_2O is most conveniently measured by using 6-l
erlenmeyer flasks calibrated to contain 6 kg H_2O. The EDTA
and NaOH may be replaced by the molar equivalent of the diso-
dium salt of EDTA.

To prepare the solution, dissolve the NaOH in about
3 l H_2O and add the EDTA and $Na_2B_4O_7 \cdot 10H_2O$. Separately,
dissolve the Na_2HPO_4 in about 400 ml H_2O over heat. Add
the dissolved components to a 20-l container. Dissolve the
SLS (270 g in about 4 l H_2O) and add to the container. The
EGME is added as necessary to control the foam. Add the
remaining H_2O and EGME to the container and mix well. The
following day, check the pH of the solution. It should be
in the range of 6.9 to 7.1 and can be adjusted if necessary
by the addition of NaOH or HCl.

Acid Detergent Solution. The following will make about 18 l acid detergent solution.

Sulfuric acid, A.R. 1N	18.0 l
Cetyltrimethylammounium bromide	
technical grade (Bromat®)	360.0 g

Prepare 1N H_2SO_4 (.99 to 1.01), most conveniently from 72% H_2SO_4 (24N) and dissolve the CTAB in the acid.

72% Sulfuric Acid. 72% sulfuric acid has a normality of 24 (12 molar) and a specific gravity of 1.634. One liter of 72% H_2SO_4 will contain 1176.96 H_2SO_4 (12 x 98.08). Since concentrated H_2SO_4 contains some H_2O, the amount of concentrated acid needed will be 1176.96 g divided by the assay reported on the bottle. The amount of H_2O required to dilute the concentrated acid to 72% will be 1634 g minus the calculated amount of concentrated acid needed. It is more convenient to make 72% H_2SO_4 in 2-l quantities to have an adequate supply available.

Weigh the amount of H_2O required into a tared 2-l MCA volumetric flask. (Tare once and etch the tare on the flask.) Place the flask in a sink and add the H_2SO_4 slowly with caution. Cool the flask and contents with running tap water. When the contents of the flask weigh 3268 g, cool the flask to 20°C and check for correct volume. The meniscus should be within 0.5 cm of the calibration mark. If the volume is too small, remove 1.5 ml and add 2.5 ml H_2O (or multiples thereof); if too large, remove 5.0 ml and add 4.45 ml H_2SO_4 (or multiple thereof). Cool, recheck weight and volume.

Asbestos. Long-fibered, purified, acid-washed asbestos, as purchased, is unsuitable for detergent fiber analysis. Before use, it should be rewashed in about 20NH_2SO_4 (technical grade) for about 2 hr, thoroughly washed with water to remove the fine particles, and ashed at 800°C for 16 hr. Used asbestos can be rewashed, ashed, and reused.

Saturated Permanganate Solution. The following will
make about 18 1 saturated permanganate solution.

Distilled water	18.0 1
Potassium permanganate, A.R.	900.0 g
Silver sulfate, A.R.	0.9 g

Dissolve the $KMnO_4$ and Ag_2SO_4 in the water. The solution must be kept out of direct sunlight. The Ag_2SO_4 acts as
a dehalogenating agent.

Buffer Solution for Permanganate Lignin Determination. The following will make about 12 1 buffer solution
for permanganate lignin determination.

Distilled water	1.2 1
Ferric nitrate nonahydrate, A.C.S.	72.0 g
Silver nitrate, A.R.	1.8 g
Acetic acid, glacial, A.C.S.	6.0 1
Potassium acetate, A.R.	60.0 g
Tertiary butyl alcohol, A.C.S.	4.8 1

Dissolve the $Fe(NO_3)_3.9H_2O$ and $AgNO_3$ in the distilled
water. Add the CH_3COOH and $KC_2H_3O_2$ and dissolve. Add the
tertiary $CH_3(CH_2)_3OH$ and mix.

Demineralizing Solution. The following will make
about 12 1 demineralizing solution.

95% Ethyl alcohol	8.4 1
Oxalic acid dihydrate, A.C.S.	600.0 g
Hydrochloric acid (12N), A.C.S.	600.0 ml
Distilled water	3.0 1

Dissolve the $(CO_2H)_2.2H_2O$ in the 95% C_2H_5OH. Add the
HCl and H_2O. Mix.

80% Ethyl Alcohol. The following will make about 10 1.

95% Ethyl alcohol	8.45 1
Distilled water	1.55 1

Mix.

Cleaning Solution for Crucibles. The following will
make about 2 l cleaning solution for crucibles.

Distilled water	2.0 l
Disodium ethylene tetra-	
acetate dehydrate, A.R.	10.0 g
Trisodium phosphate, A.R.	100.0 g
Potassium hydroxide, A.C.S.	400.0 g

Dissolve the $Na_2EDTA.2H_2O$, Na_3PO_4 and KOH in the H_2O.
The solution is very caustic. Rubber gloves and eye protection should be used when handling it.

B.   Procedures

Cell Wall (dietary fiber) Determination. The cell
wall contains the hemicelluloses, cellulose, and lignin,
with some fiber-bound protein.

1.   Weigh up to 0.5 g of the air-dry sample, ground
to pass a 1-mm screen, into a beaker. Add, with a calibrated scoop, about 0.5 g sodium sulfite anhydrous (Na_2SO_3).
Add about 100 ml neutral detergent solution. Heat to boiling in 5 to 6 min. Adjust heat to give an even boil and
reflux for 1 hr. Allow 3 min between each determination.

2.   Place tared Gooch crucibles on the filter manifold.
Remove beaker, swirl to suspend the cell walls, and fill the
crucible. Using minimal vacuum, start the filtering process.
At no time should the beaker contents be added to an empty
crucible under vacuum. Increase the vacuum as needed to
achieve filtration. Rinse the sample into the crucible with
a minimum of hot water. The hot water should be 90 to 100°C.
Wash the sample at least twice with hot water. Wash twice
with acetone, A.R., and suck dry. Dry the crucibles for
8 hr or overnight at 100°C in the forced-air oven and weigh
to obtain the yield of cell wall. Ash the crucibles and
contents at 500°C for a minimum of 3 hr, remove to the oven,
and weigh. The loss in weight on ashing is the organic cell
wall.

The most common problem encountered in running cell-
wall determinations is difficulty in filtration, usually the
result of technique. The refluxed sample should never be

added to an empty crucible under vacuum. Only when sample
has been added to the crucible should filtration be started,
and then under a minimum of vacuum. The suction force should
be increased only when the filtration slows. A compromise
sometimes has to be made between the cooling of the crucible
contents and the vacuum force, but this can be overcome by
reducing the amount of sample added to the crucible. If the
filtration ceases, back pressure should be applied to the
crucible and contents to remove the fiber blocking the pores.
However, there can be filtration difficulties because of the
composition of the cell contents, e.g., protein, starch, mucilages, and gums.

When it is suspected that high levels of protein are
hindering filtration, a protease compatible with detergents
may be used. The protease is added to the beaker containing
the sample and ND solution, and the contents are allowed to
incubate overnight in a warm place before refluxing and filtering (61). Sometimes using filter paper instead of crucibles helps (50), and a nitrogen determination can be made on
the residue. King and Tavener (42) have suggested a 2-hr
reflux time, although with longer reflux times there is a
danger of excessive Maillard reactions occurring.

High levels of starch will interfere in filtration,
especially as the crucible contents cool and the starch
comes out of solution. The addition of a bacterial α-amylase
to the crucible and contents should improve filtration (44),
but Van Soest has found that detergents destroy the $1 \rightarrow 6$
activity of these enzymes. He has proposed a tentative cell-
wall procedure for samples high in starch (61), in which the
sample is refluxed for 30 min in 50 ml of ND solution to
solubilize the starch. Then, add 50 ml of cold ND solution
and 2 ml of a 2% solution of the enzyme in water, and return
the beaker to the reflux unit without adjusting the heat
until 60 min have elapsed since the commencement of the initial boiling. Filter the sample and wash with hot water.
Triturate the fiber matt with a glass rod and 2 ml of the
enzyme solution and add about 30 ml of 70 to 80°C water.
After stirring, let stand for a few minutes; then filter
and wash twice with hot water and twice with acetone.

Some materials contain a high concentration of gums
and mucilages. When these materials are refluxed in ND solution, unfilterable gels are produced. In these cases, the

best estimate of cell wall may be through a protein correction on the ammonium oxalate or 80% ethyl alcohol residues (56). These estimates will include the mucilages and
gums that are not normally considered to be part of the cell
wall since, similar to the pectins, they are highly digestible in the rumen. There is no problem in conducting an ADR
determination on these materials. It may be necessary to use
extensive acid hydrolysis and chromatography to estimate the
cell wall of these materials.

Acid Detergent Residue. The acid detergent residue
contains the lignin, cutin, cellulose, and silica. It is
primarily a step in the determination of lignin.

1.   Weigh 1 g air-dry sample, ground to pass a 1-mm
screen, into a beaker. Add 100 ml acid detergent solution,
bring to the boil in 5 to 6 min, adjust heat to a steady
boil, and reflux for 1 hr.

2.   Place previously tared Gooch crucibles on the
filter manifold. Filter the samples using the same procedure
as described for cell walls. More than two washes with hot
water may be necessary to remove all the acid. Wash twice
with acetone or until all color is removed and suck dry.
Lumping of the residue may occur and will create problems
in the subsequent lignin determination. If lumping occurs,
the residue may be washed with hexanes. Dry for 8 hr or
overnight at 100°C and weigh. The yield is the acid detergent residue.

Unless a material contains no hemicelluloses, the ADR
value should always be less than that of the cell wall, once
corrections for ash are made. However, on occasion, the ADR
value may be substantially greater. In forages, especially
from tropical areas, this is most commonly due to the effect
of the detergent solutions on silica. The acid detergent
solution recovers all the silica in the residue, but silica
is variably soluble in neutral detergent solution. If silica
is the problem, the cell-wall value should be corrected for
the dissolved silica by running silica determinations on both
the ND and AD residues.

A more frequent cause of anomalous ADR values is the
precipitation in acid solutions of organic compounds that
are soluble in neutral detergent solution. Tannins and

aspergellic acid are such compounds. Pectic substances,
soluble in neutral detergent solution, can be precipitated
in the ADR (4). To correct for these precipitates, sequential analysis may be applied in which the ADR determination
is conducted on a sample previously extracted with neutral
detergent solution. A problem arises in doing sequential
analyses in that lignin (29) and cutin are partially solubilized when Na_2SO_3 is added in the NDR determination.
Sodium sulfite is included in the standard cell-wall procedure to increase the removal of protein (71), and its
use in that analysis should be retained, since the loss
of lignin does not compensate for the incomplete removal
of protein; however, it should be excluded in sequential
analysis.

Hemicelluloses. A presumptive analysis for the hemicelluloses may be obtained by subtracting the acid detergent
residue yield from that of the cell wall. This may be refined by taking into account the ash, nitrogen, lignin, and
cutin differences which may occur in the acid detergent
residue and cell wall. The sequential analysis, starting
with a cell-wall determination without the addition of
Na_2SO_3 followed by an acid detergent residue analysis, may
be the best estimator of the hemicellulose content.

72% Sulfuric Acid Lignin. This analysis should be conducted at 20 to 22°C.

1. Prepare the acid detergent residue.

2. Place the crucibles containing the ADR in an
enamelled pan. Add an amount of acid-washed asbestos about
equal in volume to the acid detergent residue and mix asbestos
and residue with a glass rod (cut several rods, about 3 in.
long, from 5/16 in. glass rod). Leave the glass rod in the
crucible and cover the contents with 72% H_2SO_4. Stir and then
fill the crucible about 3/4 full with 72% H_2SO_4. Thereafter,
at hourly intervals, fill the crucibles with 72% H_2SO_4 and
stir. When 3 hr have elapsed from the initial addition of
72% H_2SO_4, filter off the acid, using the filter manifold
and vacuum. Wash with hot water until free from acid, rinse,
and remove the glass rod. Dry at 100°C for 8 hr or overnight
and weigh.

Permanganate Lignin, Cellulose, Silica, and Cutin. This
analysis should be conducted at 20 to 25°C.

1.   Prepare acid detergent residue.

2.   Mix saturated permanganate solution and permanganate lignin buffer solution in the ratio of 2:1 by volume,
allowing about 40 ml of the combined solution per determination. The mixed solution is stable for about 1 day only.

3.   Place the crucibles containing the ADR in an
enameled pan. Add cold water to the pan to a level short
of the sinter glass plate so as not to wet the ADR. Add
about 20 to 25 ml of the combined solution to each crucible,
then more water to the pan to restrict the flow of solution
from the crucibles. With glass rods, mix the contents of
the crucibles to wet thoroughly all particles. Leave rods
in the crucibles. Add further combined solution to the
crucibles to about 2/3 full, and adjust the water level.
Allow the crucibles to stand for 90 ± 15 min, stirring occasionally. The solution should remain purple for the duration
of the delignification step. If the solution turns pink to
brown, it indicates that the permanganate is exhausted. The
exhausted solution should be sucked off and fresh solution
added. This will occur only in samples high in lignin. On
the other hand, in samples low in lignin, especially immature
plant material, there is the danger of cellulosic carbohydrates being lost and, in this case, the flow of the combined
solution must be severely restricted.

After 90 min, using the filtering manifold, suck off
the solution, and place the crucibles in a clean pan. Add
about 20 ml demineralizing solution to each crucible. Foam-
ing may occur and care has to be taken to avoid spillage.
After about 5 min, filter off the solution, refill with about
20 ml, and stir to mix well. Rinse the sides of the crucibles
with the solution. Two treatments with demineralizing solution are usually sufficient, although a third may be necessary. Demineralization will normally take from 30 to 60 min.
The delignification is complete when the fiber in the crucible
is white to grey in color (the color of the cellulose, depending on the substrate), and there are no black particles.
There may be brown particles of cutin. Suck off all the demineralizing solution, wash twice with 80% ethyl alcohol,
rinsing and removing the glass rods on the second 80% alcohol

wash, and wash twice with acetone. Suck dry, place in an
oven at 100°C for 8 hr or overnight, and weigh. The loss
in weight from the ADR is the permanganate lignin.

4.   If no cutin is present, the crucible and residue
can be ashed at 500°C for 3 hr, cooled to 100°C, and weighed.
The loss in weight on ashing is an estimate of the cellulose.

5.   Certain plant materials may be high in silica.
A presumptive analysis for silica may be made by treating
the ash with 48% hydrobromic acid (HBr). The ash is wetted
with HBr (no more than 4 ml per sample) and allowed to stand
for 1 to 2 hr. Then suck off the HBr, wash twice with acetone, and ash briefly at 500°C. Cool to 100°C and weigh.
The weight of ash remaining in the crucible is an estimate
of silica.

6.   Cutin resists oxidation by $KMnO_4$ and hydrolysis
by 72% H_2SO_4. If substantial amounts of cutin are present,
as in seed hulls, the sulfuric acid lignin analysis would
include the cutin in the lignin fraction. If using the permanganate lignin procedure, the cutin would be included in
the cellulose estimate. Thus, a cutin determination may be
necessary.

After completing step 3 in the permanganate lignin
procedure, treat the residue with 72% H_2SO_4 as in the sulfuric acid lignin method, but omit the asbestos. Dry the
crucible and contents at 100°C for 8 hr or overnight and
weigh. The loss in weight is an estimate of cellulose.
Then ash at 500°C for 3 hr, cool to 100°C, and weigh. The
loss in weight on ashing is an estimate of the cutin.

Acid Detergent Nitrogen

1.   Prepare acid detergent residue as above, but use
a 2-g sample and filter on Whatman #54 paper using vacuum.

2.   Analyze the ADR for nitrogen (N) content, and
express the result either as N or N x 6.25 in the initial
sample dry matter.

Heat-drying of feedstuffs and feces at temperatures
above 50 to 55°C frequently results in analytically significant increases in the cell wall, acid detergent residue, and
lignin. This increased yield is mainly due to the production

of artifact lignin via the Maillard reaction (nonenzymatic browning), in which carbohydrates and proteins condense to form an insoluble polymer (24, 26, 64). Maillard products may be deliberately produced to impart flavor to some foods.

The carbohydrates may be simple sugars (furanosides are more reactive than pyranosides) or polysaccharides. Hemicelluloses are fairly reactive but cellulose and starch much less so. Ascorbic acid will react. It is the free amino groups in the amino acids and proteins that participate in the condensation; thus lysine is very susceptible. Unsaturated lipids can be part of the Maillard complex. Water is a catalyst in the reaction. Artifact lignin may also be produced using a microwave oven as a method of drying forages (15).

When heat damage has occurred or is expected in a sample, the artifact lignin can be estimated by running a nitrogen determination on the acid detergent residue (25, 64) and applying the value to a correction equation, as follows:

$$L_C = 1.208 \ L_o - 10.75 \ N_o + 0.42$$

where L_C = corrected lignin ($72\% \ H_2SO_4$)

L_o = observed lignin ($72\% \ H_2SO_4$)

N_o = amount of nitrogen in the acid detergent residue expressed on a whole-sample basis

or

$$L_C = 1.10 \ L_o - 7.6 \ N_o + 0.3$$

where L_C = corrected lignin ($KMnO_4$)

L_o = observed lignin ($KMnO_4$)

N_o = amount of nitrogen in the acid detergent residue expressed on a whole-sample basis

and

Artifact lignin = $L_o - L_C$

Corrected ADR = observed ADR − artifact lignin

The protein in the Maillard complex is not digested by
the enzymes proliferated by the mammalian tract; neither is
it made available through lower-gut fermentation. This
fiber-bound protein may be very significant in certain cooked
foods. In evaluating these foods for protein content, the
unavailable protein should be accounted for by analyzing for
the nitrogen bound in the acid detergent residue.

Acid detergent nitrogen analysis has been applied in
digestion studies (46, 49) to fractionate the fecal nitrogen
into that associated with the feed and that of metabolic
(endogenous plus microbial) origin. The fecal nitrogen insoluble in acid detergent solution comes from the diet. If
the feces are contaminated with hair, the ADN will overesti-
mate the residual feed nitrogen since hair proteins are
insoluble in acid detergent solution, but that nitrogen which
is solubilized will be the best estimator of metabolic nitrogen. Hair proteins are solubilized in neutral detergent when
sodium sulfite is included. Thus, to estimate the true digestibility of food proteins, the fecal cell-wall nitrogen
should be measured.

Cleaning Crucibles

1. Make a suction device by boring a hole in a No. 12
rubber stopper and inserting one end of a 50-ml pipette in
the hole. Connect the other end of the pipette to a vacuum
source through a suitable trap (1- or 2-1 filtering flask).

2. Place the ashed, water-washed crucibles in an
enameled pan, add about 50 ml of the cleaning solution to
each crucible, and heat pan and contents over a steam bath
for about 15 min. Using the suction device, suck the cleaning solution back into the crucible until about 2/3 full.
Allow the solution to filter through. Repeat. Then wash
the crucibles under hot tap water to remove all traces of
alkali, and finally wash the crucibles in distilled water.

The cleaning solution is very caustic and rubber gloves
and eye protection should be worn. Excessive cleaning will
cause rapid deterioration of the sinter glass plate. Cleaning should not take more than 1 hr. Uden (60) has had success
using an ultrasonic bath for cleaning clogged crucibles.

Generally, the ingredients of the diet for humans in the Western hemisphere are low in fiber and high in soluble carbohydrates, protein, and fat, which makes cell-wall analyses difficult. It may be more feasible to remove the interfering substances from a large sample of the food to be analyzed and do the detergent procedures on the extracted residue.

VII. CONCLUSIONS

With the increasing interest in dietary fiber and its implications in gastrointestinal disease, the evaluation of foods on a fiber basis is desirable. The crude fiber method fails to recover a variable proportion of the plant structural carbohydrates and lignin. Elaborate fractionation methods to separate and measure the various sugar and polysaccharide fractions can be tedious and time consuming. The detergent system of fiber analysis has been widely accepted in the animal nutrition field and does have a nutritional basis. It is rapid and will allow the screening of a wide spectrum of foods.

REFERENCES

1. Arroyo-Aguilu, J. A., and Evans, J. L., 1972, Nutrient digestibility of low-fiber rations in the ruminant animal, J. Dairy Sci., 55:1266.

2. Association of Official Analytical Chemists, Official Methods of Analysis of the Association of Official Analytical Chemists, XI edition, AOAC, Washington, DC, 1970.

3. Bailey, R. W., 1964, Pasture quality and ruminant nutrition. Carbohydrate composition of ryegrass varieties grown as sheep pastures, N. Z. J. Agric. Res., 7:496.

4. Bailey, R. W., and Ulyatt, M. J., 1970, Pasture quality and ruminant nutrition, II. Carbohydrates and lignin composition of detergent-extracted residues from pasture grasses and legumes, N. Z. J. Agric. Res., 13:591.

5. Bevenue, A., and Williams, K. T., 1959, Note on the
    use of detergents for removal of nitrogen from plant
    materials, J. A. O. A. C., 42:441.

6. Blake, J. D., and Richards, G. N., 1970a, Polysaccha-
    rides of tropical pasture herbage, I. Studies on the
    distribution of the major polysaccharide components
    of spear grass (Heteropogon Contortus) during growth,
    Aust. J. Chem., 23:2353.

7. Blake, J. D., and Richards, G. N., 1970b, Polysaccha-
    rides of tropical pasture herbage, II. A xylan from
    the leaf of spear grass (Heteropogon Contortus),
    Aust. J. Chem., 23:2361.

8. Bryant, M. P., 1974, Nutritional features and ecology
    of predominant anaerobic bacteria of the intestinal
    tract, 27:1313.

9. Burkitt, D. P., 1973, Epidemiology of large bowel
    disease: the role of fibre, Proc. Nutr. Soc., 32:145.

10. Burkitt, D. P., and Trowell, H. C., Refined Carbohy-
    drate Foods and Disease: Some Implications of Dietary
    Fibre (London: Academic Press, 1975).

11. Butterworth, M. H., 1967, The digestibility of tropical
    grasses, Nutr. Abstr. Rev., 37:349.

12. Crampton, E. W., Irwin, M. I., Lloyd, L. E., and
    Neilsen, H. R., 1951, The apparent digestibility of
    essentially similar diets by rats, guinea pigs, sheep,
    swine and by human subjects, J. Nutr., 43:541.

13. Crampton, E. W., and Maynard, L. A., 1938, The relation
    of cellulose and lignin content to the nutritive value
    of animal feeds, J. Nutr., 15:383.

14. Cummings, J. W., 1973, Progress report - dietary fibre,
    Gut, 14:69.

15. Darah, C., Personal communication.

16. Eastwood, M. A., 1973, Vegetable fibre: its physical
    properties, Proc. Nutr. Soc., 32:137.

17. Farrell, D. J., 1973, Digestibility by pigs of the major chemical components of diets high in plant cell-wall constituents, Animal Production, 16:43.

18. Fonnesbeck, P. V., 1968, Digestion of soluble and fibrous carbohydrate of forages by horses, J. Animal Sci., 27:1336.

19. Fonnesbeck, P. V., 1969, Partitioning the nutrients of forage for horses, J. Animal Sci., 28:624.

20. Fonnesbeck, P. V., Harris, L. E., and Kearl, L. C., 1974, Digestion of plant cell walls by animals, abstract, J. Animal Sci., 39:182.

21. Foster, J. F., Yang, J. T., and Yui, N. H., 1950, Extraction and electrophoretic analyses of the proteins of corn, Cereal Chem., 27:477.

22. Gaillard, B. D. E., 1962, The relationship between cell-wall constituents of roughage and the digestibility of the organic matter, J. Agric. Sci., Camb., 59:369.

23. Gall, L. S., 1970, Normal fecal flora of man, Am. J. Clin. Nutr., 23:1457.

24. Goering, H. K., Gordon, C. H., Hemken, R. W., Waldo, D. R., Van Soest, P. J., and Smith, L. W., 1972, Analytical estimates of nitrogen digestibility in heat-damaged forages, J. Dairy Sci., 55:1275.

25. Goering, H. K., and Van Soest, P. J., Forage fiber analyses (apparatus, reagents, procedures, and some applications), Agr. Handbook No. 379, A. R. S., USDA, Washington, D. C., 1970.

26. Goering, H. K., Van Soest, P. J., and Hemken, R. W., 1973, Relative susceptibility of forages to heat damage as affected by moisture, temperature and pH, J. Dairy Sci., 56:137.

27. Groen, J. J., 1973, Why bread in the diet lowers serum cholesterol, Proc. Nutr. Soc., 32:159.

28. Harkin, J. M., "Lignin," in: Chemistry and Biochemistry of Herbage, G. W. Butler and R. W. Bailey, editors, Vol. 1 (New York: Academic Press, 1973) p. 323.

29. Hartley, R. D., 1972, p-Coumaric and ferulic acid components of cell walls of ryegrass and their relationships with lignin and digestibility, J. Sci. Fd. Agric., 23:1347.

30. Hellendoorn, E. W., Noordhoff, M. G., and Slagman, J., 1975, Enzymatic determination of the indigestible residue (dietary fibre) content of human foods, J. Sci. Fd. Agric., 26:1461.

31. Hill, M. J., 1974, Bacteria and the etiology of colonic cancer, Cancer, 34:815.

32. Hintz, H. F., Argenzio, R. A., and Schryver, H. F., 1971, Digestion coefficients, blood glucose levels and molar percentage of volatile acids in intestinal fluid of ponies fed varying forage-grain ratios, J. Animal Sci., 33:992.

33. Hintz, H. F., Hogue, D. E., Walker Jr., E. F., Lowe, J. E., and Schryver, H. F., 1971, Apparent digestion in various segments of the digestive tract of ponies fed diets with varying roughage-grain ratios, J. Animal Sci., 32:245.

34. Hintz, H. F., Schryver, H. F., and Halbert, M., 1973, A note on the comparison of digestion by new world camels, sheep and ponies, Animal Production, 16:303.

35. Holdeman, L. V., Good, I. J., and Moore, W. E. C., 1976, Human fecal flora: variation in bacterial composition within individuals and a possible effect on emotional stress, Appl. Env. Microb., 31:359.

36. Hoover, W. H., and Clarke, S. D., 1972, Fiber digestion in the beaver, J. Nutr., 102:9.

37. Hoppert, C. A., and Clark, A. J., 1945, Digestibility and effect on laxation of crude fiber and cellulose in certain common foods, J. Amer. Diet Assn., 21:157.

38.   Hummel, F. C., Shepherd, M. I., and Macy, I. G., 1943,
      Disappearance of cellulose and hemicellulose from the
      digestive tracts of children, J. Nutr., 25:59.

39.   Jones, A. S., 1953, The isolation of bacterial nuclei
      acids using cetyl trimethyl ammonium (Cetavlon),
      Biochim. Biophys. Acta., 10:607.

40.   Keys Jr., J. E., and Van Soest, P. J., 1970, Digesti-
      bility of forages by the meadow vole (Microtus pennsyl-
      vanicus), J. Dairy Sci., 53:1502.

41.   Keys Jr., J. E., Van Soest, P. J., and Young, E. P.,
      1969, Comparative study of the digestibility of forage
      cellulose and heimcellulose in ruminants and non-
      ruminants, J. Animal Sci., 29:11.

42.   King, R. H., and Taverner, M. R., 1975, Prediction of
      the digestible energy in pig diets from analyses of
      fibre contents, Animal Production, 21:275.

43.   Lucas Jr., H. L., Smart Jr., W. W. G., Cipolloni, M. A.,
      and Gross, H. D., 1961, Relations between digestibility
      and composition of feeds and foods, S-45 Report,
      North Carolina State College (mimeo).

44.   McQueen, R. E., Personal communication.

45.   McQueen, R. E., and Van Soest, P. J., 1975, Fungal
      cellulase and hemicellulase prediction of forage
      digestibility, J. Dairy Sci., 58:1482.

46.   Mason, V. C., 1969, Some observations on the distribu-
      tion and origin of nitrogen in sheep faeces, J. Agric.
      Sci. Camb., 73:99.

47.   Mertens, D. R., Application of theoretical mathematical
      models to cell wall digestion and forage intake in
      ruminants, Ph.D. Thesis, Cornell Univ., Ithaca, N. Y.

48.   Raymond, T. L., Connor, W. E., Robertson, J. B., and
      Van Soest, P. J., October 1976, Measurement of dietary
      fiber balance in man, Circulation, supplement.

49.   Robertson, J. B., and Van Soest, P. J., 1975, A note
      on digestibility in sheep as influenced by level of
      intake, Animal Production, 21:89.

50.   Robertson, J. B., Van Soest, P. J., and Torres, F.,
      1972, Substitution of filter paper for crucibles in
      the in vitro true digestibility determination, J. Dairy
      Sci., 55:1305.

51.   Salo, M. L., 1965, Determination of carbohydrate frac-
      tions in animal foods and faeces, Acta Agric. Fenn.,
      105:1.

52.   Southgate, D. A. T., 1969a, Determination of carbohy-
      drates in foods, I. Available carbohydrate, J. Sci.
      Fd. Agric., 20:326.

53.   Southgate, D. A. T., 1969b, Determination of carbohy-
      drates in foods, II. Unavailable carbohydrates, J. Sci.
      Fd. Agric., 20:331.

54.   Southgate, D. A. T., and Durnin, J. V. G. A., 1970,
      Calorie conversion factors. An experimental reassess-
      ment of the factors used in the calculation of the
      energy value of human diets, Brit. J. Nutr., 24:517.

55.   Spiller, G. A., and Amen, R. J., 1975, Dietary fiber
      in human nutrition, Crit. Rev. in Fd. Sci. and Nutr.,
      7:39.

56.   Sullivan, J. T., 1964, The chemical composition of
      forages in relation to digestibility by ruminants,
      ARS 34-62, Agricultural Research Council, USDA,
      Washington, D. C.

57.   Tilley, J. M. A., and Terry, R. A., 1963, A two-stage
      technique for the in vitro digestion of forage crops,
      J. Brit. Grassland Soc., 18:104.

58.   Trowell, H., 1973, Dietary Fibre. Ischaemic heart
      disease and diabetes mellitus, Proc. Nutr. Soc., 32:151.

59.   Tyler, C., 1975, Albrecht Thaer's hay equivalents:
      fact or fiction, Nutrition Abstracts and Reviews, 45:1.

60.   Uden, P., Personal communication.

61.   Van Soest, P. J., Personal communication.

62.   Van Soest, P. J., 1963a, Use of detergents in the
      analysis of fibrous feeds, I. Preparation of fiber
      residues of low nitrogen content, J. A. O. A. C.,
      46:825.

63.   Van Soest, P. J., 1963b, Use of detergents in the
      analysis of fibrous feeds, II. A rapid method for
      the determination of fiber and lignin, J. A. O. A. C.,
      46:829.

64.   Van Soest, P. J., 1965, Use of detergents in the analy-
      sis of fibrous feeds, III. Study of effects of heating
      and drying on yield of fiber and lignin in forages,
      J. A. O. A. C., 48:785.

65.   Van Soest, P. J., 1966, Nonnutritive residues: A system
      of analysis for the replacement of crude fiber, J. A.
      O. A. C., 49:546.

66.   Van Soest, P. J., 1967, Development of a comprehensive
      system of feed analyses and its application to forages,
      J. Animal Sci., 26:119.

67.   Van Soest, P. J., 1968, Structural and chemical
      characteristics which limit the nutritive value of
      forages. In: Forage: economics-quality, Amer. Soc.
      of Agronomy, Spec. Publ. No. 13, p. 63.

68.   Van Soest, P. J., 1975, Physico-chemical aspects of
      fibre digestion, Proc. IV, International Symposium
      on Ruminant Physiology, I. W. McDonald and A. C. I.
      Warner, Sydney, Australia, pp. 351.

69.   Van Soest, P. J., and McQueen, R. E., 1973, The chem-
      istry and estimation of fibre, Proc. Nutr. Soc., 32:123.

70.   Van Soest, P. J. and Moore, L. A., 1965, New chemical
      methods for analysis of forages for the purpose of
      predicting nutritive value, Proc. IX, International
      Grassland Congress, p. 783.

71.   Van Soest, P. J., and Wine, R. H., 1967, Use of
      detergents in the analysis of fibrous feeds, IV.
      Determination of plant cell-wall constituents,
      J. A. O. A. C., 50:50.

72.   Van Soest, P. J., and Wine, R. H., 1968, Determination
      of lignin and cellulose in acid-detergent fiber with
      permanganate, J. A. O. A. C., 51:780.

73.   Van Soest, P. J., Wine, R. H., and Moore, L. A., 1966,
      Estimation of the true digestibility of forages by
      the in vitro digestion of cell walls, Proc. X,
      International Grassland Congress, p. 438.

74.   Visek, W. J., 1974, Some biochemical considerations
      in utilization of nonspecific nitrogen, J. Agr. Food
      Chem., 22:174.

75.   Visek, W. J. and Roberton, J. B., 1973, Dried brewers
      grains in dog diets, Proc. Cornell Nutrition Conf.,
      p. 40.

76.   Waldo, D. R., 1969, Factors influencing the voluntary
      intake of forages, Proc. Nat. Conf. Forage Quality
      Evaluation and Utilization, Lincoln, Nebraska, p. E1.

77.   Waldo, D. R., Smith, L. W., and Cox, E. L., 1972,
      Model of cellulose disappearance from the rumen,
      J. Diary Sci., 55:125.

78.   Williams, K. T., and Bevenue, A., 1956, Problems and
      techniques in the analysis of plant material for hemi-
      cellulose, J. A. O. A. C., 39:901.

79.   Williams, R. D., and Olmsted, W. H., 1936, The effect
      of cellulose, hemicellulose, and lignin on the weight
      of the stool: A contribution to the study of laxation
      in man, J. Nutr., 11:433.

80.   Wrick, K., 1976, Personal communication.

CHAPTER 2

WHEAT BRAN: COMPOSITION AND DIGESTIBILITY

Robert M. Saunders

Agricultural Research Service
U.S. Department of Agriculture

Berkeley, California

I. INTRODUCTION

Studies have shown that feeding wheat bran to humans often results in therapeutic improvement in lower alimentary tract disorders (10, 26, 27). The actual component(s) of bran responsible for these clinical observations has not been determined, although the indigestible constituents (or dietary fiber) presumably play an important role. Little is known of the chemistry of the many cellular layers that comprise bran. Studies relating to the various components of bran and their fate during digestion are reviewed.

II. MORPHOLOGY OF BRAN (16)

Wheat produces dry, one-seeded fruits. The seed consists of germ, or embryo, and endosperm, enclosed by a nucellar epidermis and a seed coat (Figure 1). This type of structure, usually called a grain or kernel or caryopsis, is characteristic of the grass family (Gramineae). The pericarp is 45 to 50 µ thick and is composed of many layers. These are, in order from the exterior to the seed, epidermis, hypodermis, intermediate cells, cross cells, and tube cells.

The outer pericarp (or beeswing) is composed of the epidermis and hypodermis, and is approximately 34 µ thick. The epidermis consists of a single layer of cells, whereas the hypodermis though usually one layer, sometimes contains two

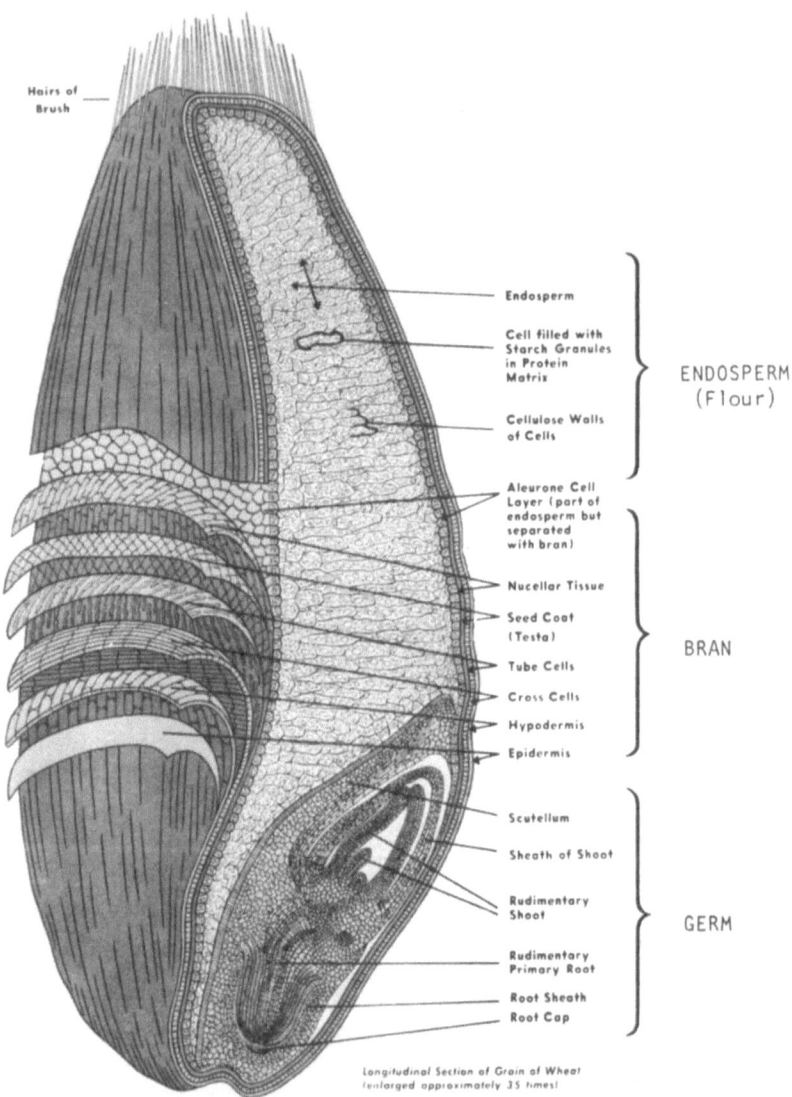

Figure 1.   Longitudinal section of kernel of wheat.
Reproduced with permission, Wheat Flour Institute,
Chicago, Illinois.

layers. The cells of both the epidermis and hypodermis have
thickened walls; thicknesses of 3 to 5.7 μ have been reported.

The intermediate cells, cross cells, and tube cells
compromise the inner pericarp. The cross cells, which
have their long axes perpendicular to the long axis of the
kernel, have dimensions of 100 to 150 μ by 15 to 20 μ with
cell walls 5 to 7 μ thick. The tube cells are cylindrical,
with their axes parallel to the long axis of the kernel.
Their dimensions are 120 to 300 μ by 12 to 15 μ.

Proceeding toward the center of the kernel the next
layer is the seed coat. This is composed of a thick outer
cuticle, a color layer, and a thin inner cuticle. The seed
coat is cutinized.

The nucellar epidermis (or hyaline layer) is about 7 μ
thick and lies between the seed coat and the aleurone layer.
Though botanically belonging to the endosperm, during milling of wheat the aleurone layer (Figure 2) adheres to the
outer layers of the kernel and becomes part of the bran.
The aleurone layer, commonly one cell thick, is reported to
be 25 to 75 μ in thickness, varying with wheat variety,
with cell walls 6 to 8 μ thick. The walls of adjacent cells
are cemented together by noncellulosic material. There are
protoplasmic connections between adjacent cells and between
these cells and adjoining starch endosperm cells. Each cell

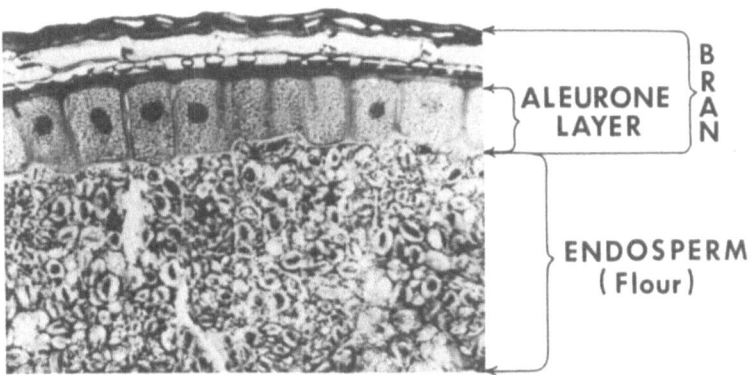

Figure 2. Cross section of wheat showing the bran fraction.

TABLE 1. Composition of Component
Parts of the Wheat Kernel[1]
(Percentages)

Outer Pericarp	Cross cells	Seed coat	Nucellar layer & seed coat	Clean bran	Starchy endosperm	Germ
2.6-4.35	0.5-1.5	0.2-1.1	2.21-3.14	11.6-21.4	74.9-86.5	0.99-3.8

[1]From data of Macmasters, Hinton, and Bradbury (16).

of the aleurone layer contains a nucleus, and a large number
of phytic acid granules (41) (so called aleurone granules or
grains) embedded in a matrix containing large quantities of
protein and fat. A breakdown of these cellular layers on a
kernel weight basis is shown in Table 1.

When wheat is milled for flour, the break occurs just
within the endosperm, close to the junction of the aleurone
layer and the endosperm (Figure 2). Thus bran contains all
the layers previously discussed above plus a small amount
of endosperm materials. Commercial wheat bran contains germ,
the matter of degree depending on the milling procedure. In
normal milling practice, the wheat is broken down into several fractions (Table 2). Commercial wheat bran refers to

TABLE 2. Commercial Milling Fractions
Derived from Whole Wheat[1]

Wheat	Bran	Shorts	Red dog	Germ	Flour
100	12.5-16.8	6.9-8.9	1.6-3.7	0.6-1.1	72.4-77.0

[1]Data from the Millfeed Manual (21).

the larger particles which are removed from the kernel.
These particles, which are platelets, range from 40 to 1600 μ

with over 90% being larger than 1500 µ, and an average
thickness of 125 µ.

III. COMPOSITION OF BRAN

The range in proximate composition of commercial bran
from different types of wheat is shown in Table 3 (21).

A. Carbohydrates

On a moisture-free basis, bran contains about 70%
carbohydrates which consists of approximately 12% starch,
8% sugars, 45% hemicelluloses[1] and 35% cellulose (9, 11).

The starch component may vary from 7% to as high as 16%
depending on the variety of wheat and degree of milling
(9, 36).

The sugars are located primarily within the aleurone
layer (40) with sucrose, raffinose and neokestose accounting
for approximately 75% of total (9, 37, 40). Other sugars
such as stachyose, fructosylraffinose, glycerol, xylose,
arabinose, glucose, fructose, and low-molecular-weight fruc-
tosans have also been reported in wheat bran (32, 37, 40).

TABLE 3. Proximate Analysis of Wheat Bran[†]
(Percentages)

Moisture	Protein (N x 6.25)	Fat	Ash	Crude fiber
3.7–17.7	11.9–22.9	3.0–6.8	3.8–9.6	6.8–17.5

†Data from the Millfeed Manual (21).

---

[1]In this text, hemicelluloses include pentosans.

There are no reported data on the composition of wheat
bran cellulose, its physical or biochemical properties.
Hemicelluloses are generally thought to be cementing tissue
(22). Bran hemicellulose, more highly branched than the
hemicelluloses of flour, straw or leaves, has as its major
component an araboxylan containing mainly L-arabinose and
D-xylose and about 10% D-glucuronic acid (1).

With the exception of the known location of the sugars
in the aleurone layer (38), very little information is available on the precise layer or layers in which the other carbohydrates are located. Bruckner (6) analyzed hand-dissected
bran layers for polysaccharides and showed the epidermis and
hypodermis were richer in hemicelluloses (50%) and crude
fiber (including cellulose) (27%) than were the cross cells
and tube cells (39 and 21% respectively). The seed coat is
known to contain cellulose and pectin (4). The cell walls
of the aleurone layer are believed to be cellulosic (5) but
cemented together with noncellulosic material.

Since approximately 12% endosperm material is generally
present in commercial bran, it should be noted that small
quantities of endosperm hemicelluloses are present. The
major sugar components of these materials are D-xylose and
L-arabinose, with smaller amounts of D-galactose and D-glucose
(42). These polysaccharides in the form of glycoproteins are
believed (9) to be responsible for the gelling power of certain wheat flour extracts. The highly branched polymers
imbibe considerable quantities of water to form solutions of
high viscosity (44). It is also likely that traces of water-
soluble β-glucans are present (28).

                              B. Lignin

Wheat bran contains less than 5% of lignin. Beeswing,
after extraction with benzene-alcohol (2:1) and 0.5% ammonium
oxelate, contained 5.6% lignin (1). The quantity of lignin
in different bran layers is not documented, nor has its
chemical composition been established.

C. Other Components

Bran contains numerous vitamins and minerals, protein (11.9 to 22.9%) and fat (3.0 to 6.8%). The vitamins include biotin, choline, folic acid, inositol, niacin, thiamine, p-aminobenzoic acid, pantothenic acid, riboflavin, and tocopherals (16). The minerals present include those being considered at present as being inadequate in typical U.S. diets, such as iron and zinc (0.014% and 0.02% dry basis, respectively) (16). Bran protein is high in the amino acid lysine, and though not as nutritionally adequate as casein, is superior to white flour protein (20), though the protein is of limited digestibility (Section IV). The fats are about 80% unsaturated, consisting mainly of linoleic (54%), oleic (23%), palmitic (20%), and linolenic (3%) (21). The aleurone layer is the major site of these nutrients, containing nearly all the vitamins, over 75% of the bran protein, about 90% of the fat, and 60% of the ash of whole bran (39).

The aleurone layer is also a rich source of enzymatic activity. Enzymes such as α-amylase, dipeptidase, phosphomoesterase, lipoxidase, and dehydrogenases have been identified in aleurone cells (5). An enzyme claimed to be effective in reducing hypertension in dogs (12) is present in bran. Low molecular weight proteins occur in bran which are α-amylase inhibitors, and which are physiologically active in man by effectively slowing down the rate of starch digestion (29, 33).

IV. BRAN DIGESTIBILITY[1]

Although experiments were conducted as long ago as the mid-nineteenth century on the digestibility of bran by humans, probably the most informative studies are those carried out by British workers during the Second World War. Macrae et al. in 1942 (17) fed 73% extraction flour (very close to present white flour in the U.S.) and whole wheat flour in the form of baked bread. The total caloric digestibility and protein digestibility of the white bread were 96.1% and 91.1%, whereas that of the whole wheat bread were

---

[1]Digestibility refers to dry-matter disappearance of all components combined in bran. Protein digestibility refers only to protein. Caloric digestibility refers to calories derived from sugars, starch, fat, and protein.

87.1% and 85.7%, respectively. The granularity of the flours
had no effect on digestibility. From these data and other
information provided by the authors it can be calculated
that the digestibility of the bran was approximately 40%,
and bran protein digestibility was about 65%. Other workers
(15, 19, 23) have also concluded that bran is poorly digested
by humans. McCance et al. (18), studying the rate of passage
of brown (i.e., more bran) and white bread through man's
digestive tract, showed that the transit time of the brown
bread in the stomach and small intestine was generally 1 hr
and 1.5 hr less, respectively, than that of the white bread.
The residue from the brown bread in the ileum and colon had
greater bulk than that from the white bread, and left the
colon 24 hr sooner than that from the white bread. These
authors concluded that greater bulk and malleability were the
main reasons for the more rapid transit and expulsion of the
brown bread residues.

Hickey et al. (14) have shown that human intestinal-gas
production was increased following consumption of wheat bran.

In-vivo studies with rats have documented the quantity
of indigestible residue remaining from white and whole wheat
breads, and wheat milling fractions including bran (31).
Digestibility averaged 92.4% for seven whole wheat breads,
97.6% for three white breads, and 47% for seven wheat brans,
on a dry weight basis. These data indicate mean indigestibility or dietary fiber to be 7.6% for whole wheat bread,
2.4% for white bread, and 53% for wheat bran.

Examination of the feces from different animals after
ingestion of bran indicated that the aleurone layer prevailed
in feces from rats (31), and chicks (38), but not in the
pig (34), and only limitedly in the calf (34). In all animals, all or part of the pericarp layers were present in the
feces.

Studies with humans, though limited, have indicated
that bran protein is poorly utilized (17). Chicks (38),
pigs (34), calves (34), and rats (8, 25, 35) also are unable
to completely digest the protein in bran. For example,
values for protein digestibility have ranged from 63% to
76% in studies by these workers. A linear relationship between protein digestibility and crude fiber has been established in rat feeding trials for wheat milling fractions including bran, and in baked wheat products (31).

V. FIBER VERSUS INDIGESTIBLE RESIDUE

Determination of crude fiber in foodstuffs is misleading. The figure obtained is substantially lower than dietary fiber or the sum of indigestible fragments. The accepted chemical procedure for determining crude fiber is erroneous due to the fact that the method hydrolyzes to varying degrees (7) cellulose, hemicellulose, and lignin, whereas the human during the digestive process does so very differently. The enzymes capable of degrading cellulose, hemicellulose, and lignin are not present in human gastrointestinal secretions; however, intestinal bacteria are capable of such digestion (45). Dietary fiber in wheat bran comprises indigestible polysaccharides and lignin and, in addition, portions of protein, fat, and other nutrients which are unavailable during the digestion process.

From data published by Macrae et al. (17) and Krebs and Mellanby (15), Moran and Pace (24) deduced that for every increase in the crude fiber content of cereals of 0.2% above a minimum of 0.15%, there was a decrease in digestibility of 1.1%. Recent work has certainly supported their thesis to the extent that total indigestibility or dietary fiber is considerably higher than crude fiber. Enzymatic procedures to measure dietary fiber, which do not destroy indigestible material, have yielded fiber values 2- to 5-fold higher than routine crude fiber determinations. Thomas (43) has reported for the same wheat sample a crude fiber content of 2.4% by a chemical method, but 8.5% by an enzymatic method. Hellendoorn et al. (13), using an enzymatic procedure, found dietary fiber values of 4%, 15.5%, and 56% for white bread, whole-wheat bread, and wheat bran, respectively. Robertson and Steh (30), on the other hand, found neutral detergent fiber values of 3.3% for white bread, and 14.9% for whole wheat bread. A visual representation (Figure 3) obtained after an in-vitro digestion (31) shows the indigestible residues left after digestion of equal quantities of bread. The residues from the whole wheat breads, mainly bran fragments, indicate a bulky indigestible residue in contrast to the residue from white bread.

By use of in-vivo studies with rats, Saunders (31) has derived a regression equation for dietary fiber in wheat milling fractions (bran, germ, shorts, red dog, and flour) wherein dietary fiber = 4.15 times crude fiber minus 0.27 (r, 0.996, P<0.01). The equivalent equation for wheat breads

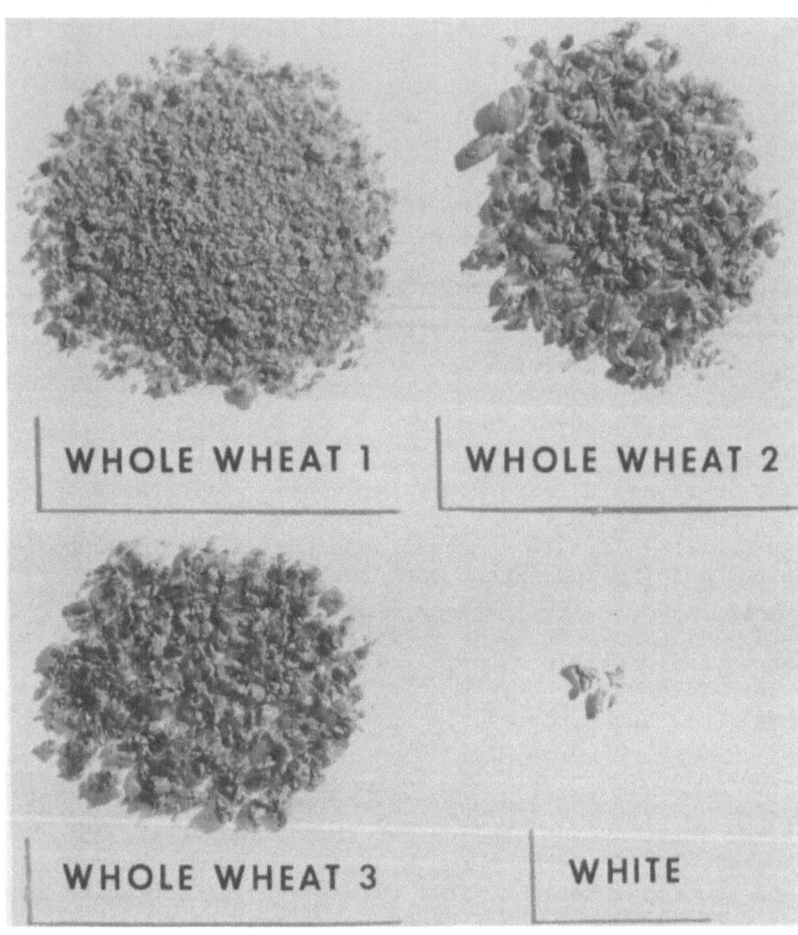

Figure 3.   Residue remaining undigested after in-vitro (35)
digestion of equal quantities of white bread and three whole-
wheat breads.

and breakfast cereals was found to be: dietary fiber = 3.43
times crude fiber + 0.78 (r, 0.836, P<0.01).

These few citations, derived from a literature in which
there are many more, deem it imperative that measurement of
dietary fiber in bran should be done with feeding tests,
by in vitro enzymatic procedures designed to duplicate a
monogastric animal, or by the neutral detergent fiber technique, once correlation with feeding trials has been established. Ideally, the analysis described by Saunders (31)
relating dietary fiber to crude fiber in rat feeding studies
should be ascertained for humans in appropriate feeding
experiments. If a similar linear relationship exists in
humans, then estimation of dietary fiber in bran and in
wheat foods will be a simple calculation based upon the traditional crude fiber measurement.

VI.   CONCLUSION

The relationship between dietary fiber and colon cancer
and heart disease is still tenuous, although definitive evidence on these interrelationships may well be forthcoming
shortly. Of the sources of foodstuffs dietary fiber, wheat
bran is one material which is receiving considerable attention. The actual dietary fiber of wheat bran is on the order
of 50 to 60%, and the physical size of bran particles is
known to be large. Not known, however, is the cellular
fraction(s) or polysaccharide(s) responsible for the therapeutic improvements. Research is needed to define wheat
bran ingestion metabolism more thoroughly before bran can
be prescribed as a beneficial food. In addition, the effects
of processing on dietary fiber, such as particle size or
cooking treatments, needs to be thoroughly studied.

ACKNOWLEDGMENT

The author thanks coworkers A. A. Betschart and D. A.
Fellers for assistance in preparation of the manuscript.

REFERENCES

1. Adams, G. A., 1955, Constitution of a hemicellulose
    from wheat bran, Can. J. Chem., 33:56.

2. Akeson, W. R., and Stahmann, M. A., 1964, Pepsin
    pancreatin digest index of protein quality evaluation,
    J. Nutr., 83:257.

3. Booth, R. G., and Moran, T., 1946, Digestibility of
    high-extraction wheat in flours, Lancet, 251:119.

4. Bradbury, D., MacMasters, M. M., and Cull, I. M.,
    1956, Structure of the mature wheat kernel, II.
    Microscopic structure of pericarp, seed coat, and
    other coverings of the endosperm and germ of hard
    red winter wheat, Cereal Chem., 33:342.

5. Bradbury, D., MacMasters, M. M., and Cull, I. M.,
    1956, Structure of the mature wheat kernel, III.
    Microscopic structure of the endosperm of hard red
    winter wheat, Cereal Chem., 33:361.

6. Bruckner, G., "Structure and composition of the
    cereal kernel," in: Bread in our Time, (Detmold,
    Germany: Moritz Schafer, 1966).

7. Cerning, J., and Guilbot, A., "Carbohydrate com-
    position of wheat, in: Wheat Production and Utiliza-
    tion, G. E. Inglett, editor, (Westport, Conn.: AVI,
    1974) p. 146.

8. Chick, M., Cutting, M. E. M., Martin, C. J., and
    Slack, E. B., 1947, Observations on the digestibility
    and nutritive value of the nitrogenous constituents
    of wheat bran, Brit. J. Nutr., 1:161.

9. D'Appolonia, B. L., Gilles, K. A., Osman, E. M., and
    Pomeranz, Y., "Carbohydrates," in: Wheat: Chemistry
    and Technology, Y. Pomeranz, editor, (St. Paul: Amer.
    Assn. of Cereal Chemists, 1971) p. 301.

10. Findley, J. M., Smith, A. N., Mitchell, W. D., Ander-
     son, A. J. B., and Eastwood, M. A., 1974, Effects of
     unprocessed bran on colon function in normal subjects
     and in diverticular disease, Lancet, 1:146.

11. Fraser, J. R., and Holmes, D. C., 1959, Proximate
     analysis of wheat flour carbohydrates, IV. Analysis
     of wholemeal flour and some of its fractions, J. Sci.
     Food Agr., 10:506.

12. Gollan, F., Richardson, E., and Goldblatt, H., 1948,
     Plant hypertensinase, J. Exp. Med., 87:29.

13. Hellendoorn, E. W., Noordhoff, M. G., and Slagman, J.,
     1975, Enzymatic determination of the indigestible
     residue (dietary fiber) content of human food, J. Sci.
     Fd. Agric., 26:1461.

14. Hickey, C. A., Murphy, E. L., and Calloway, D. H.,
     1972, Intestinal-gas production following ingestion of
     commercial wheat cereals and milling fractions, Cereal
     Chem., 49:276.

15. Krebs, H. A., and Mellanby, K., 1942, Digestibility of
     national wheat meal, Lancet, 242:319.

16. Macmasters, M. M., Hinton, J. J. C., and Bradbury, D.,
     "Microscopic structure and composition of the wheat
     kernel," in: Wheat: Chemistry and Technology, Y. Pomer-
     anz, editor, (St. Paul: Amer. Assn. of Cereal Chemists,
     1971) p. 51.

17. Macrae, T. F., Hutchinson, J. C. D., Irwin, J. O.,
     Bacon, J. S. D., and McDougall, E. I., 1942, Compara-
     tive digestibility of wholemeal and white breads and
     effect of the degree of fineness of grinding on the
     former, J. Hyg., 42:423.

18. McCance, R. A., Prior, K. M., and Widdowson, E. M.,
     1953, A radiological study of the rate of passage
     of brown and white bread through the digestive tract
     of man, Brit. J. Nutr., 7:98.

19.   McCance, R. A., and Walsham, C. M., 1946, The digesti-
      bility and absorption of the calories, proteins,
      purines, fat and calcium in wholemeal wheaten breads,
      Brit. J. Nutr., 2:26.

20.   Miladi, S., Hegsted, D. M., Saunders, R. M., and Kohler,
      G. O., 1972, The relative nutritive value, amino acid
      content, and digestibility of the proteins of wheat
      mill fractions, Cereal Chem., 49:119.

21.   Millfeed Manual, The Millers National Federation,
      Chicaco, Illinois, 1972.

22.   Montgomery, R., and Smith, F., 1952, Chemistry of the
      carbohydrates, Ann. Rev. Biochem., 21:79.

23.   Moran, T., 1959, Nutritional significance of recent
      work on wheat, flour and bread, Nutr. Abstr. Reviews,
      29:1.

24.   Moran, T., and Pace, J., 1942, Digestibility of high-
      extraction wheatmeals, Nature, 150:224.

25.   Olsen, E. M., Summers, J. D., and Slinger, S. J., 1968,
      Evaluation of protein quality in wheat by-products:
      Digestibility of protein and absorption of amino acids
      by the rat., J. Anim. Sci., 48:215.

26.   Painter, N. S., Almeida, A. Z., and Colebourne, K. W.,
      1972, Unprocessed bran in treatment of diverticular
      disease of the colon, Brit. Med. J., 2:137.

27.   Piepmeyer, J. L. , 1974, Use of unprocessed bran in
      treatment of irritable bowel syndrome, Am. J. Clin.
      Nutr., 27:106.

28.   Preece, I. A., and MacKenzie, K. G., 1952, Non-starchy
      polysaccharides of cereal grains, II. Distribution
      of water-soluble gum-like materials in cereals, J. Inst.
      Brewing, 58:457.

29.   Puls, W., and Keup, U., 1973, Influence of α-amylase
      inhibitor on blood glucose, serum insulin and NEFA
      in starch leading tests in rats, dogs, and man,
      Diabetologia, 9:97.

30. Robertson, J. B., and Steh, 1975, quoted by G. A.
     Spiller and R. J. Amen, Dietary fiber in human nutri-
     tion, Crit. Rev. Food Sci. and Nutr., 7:39.

31. Saunders, R. M., October 1976, The relationship of
     dietary fiber to digestibility in cereal milling
     fractions, 61st Annual Meeting, Amer. Assn. Cereal
     Chemists, New Orleans, Louisiana.

32. Saunders, R. M., 1971, Fructosylraffinose, a tetra-
     saccharide in wheat bran, Phytochemistry, 10:491.

33. Saunders, R. M., 1975, Alpha-amylase inhibitors in
     wheat and other cereals, Cereal Foods World, 20:282.

34. Saunders, R. M., Connor, M. A., Kohler, G. O., and
     Blaylock, L. G., 1974, Digestion of wheat bran by
     calves and pigs, J. Anim. Sci., 38:1272.

35. Saunders, R. M., and Kohler, G. O., 1972, In vitro
     determination of protein digestibility in wheat mill-
     feeds for monogastric animals, Cereal Chem., 49:98.

36. Saunders, R. M., Potter, A. L., Connor, M., McCready,
     R. M., and Walker, H. G., 1970, Analysis of starch in
     wheat milling fractions, Cereal Chem., 47:147.

37. Saunders, R. M., and Walker, H. G., 1969, The sugars
     of wheat bran, Cereal Chem., 46:85.

38. Saunders, R. M., Walker, H. G., and Kohler, G. O., 1969,
     Aleurone cells and the digestibility of wheat mill
     feeds, Poultry Sci., 43:1497.

39. Shetlar, M. R., Rankin, G. T., Lyman, J. F., and France,
     W. G., 1947, Investigation of the proximate chemical
     composition of the separate bran layers of wheat, Ce-
     real Chem., 24:111.

40. Stevens, D. J., 1970, Free sugars of wheat aleurone
     cells, J. Sci. Food Agr., 21:31.

41. Stevens, D. J., 1975, Cited in Cereal Science in the
     U. K.-Achievements and Prospects by C. T. Greenwood,
     Cereal Foods World, 20:23.

42.   Strobel, R. G., and Holme, J., 1963, Chemical compo-
       sition of the water-soluble constituents of bleached
       cake flour, Cereal Chem., $\underline{40}$:361.

43.   Thomas, B., 1972, Enzymatic procedures for the deter-
       mination of structural cell wall constituents and their
       interpretation, Intern. Assoc. for Cereal Chemistry
       Congr., Vienna.

44.   Udy, D. C., 1956, The intrinsic viscosities of the
       water-soluble components of wheat flour, Cereal Chem.,
       $\underline{33}$:67.

45.   Weinstein, L. R., Olson, R. E., Van Itallie, T. B.,
       Caso, E., Johnson, D., and Inglefinger, F. J., 1961,
       Diet as related to gastrointestinal function, J. Amer.
       Med. Assoc., $\underline{176}$:935.

CHAPTER 3

THE CHEMICAL STRUCTURE OF LIGNIN AND QUANTITATIVE

AND QUALITATIVE METHODS OF ANALYSIS IN FOODSTUFFS

Anthony J. Gordon

Department of Animal Physiology
University of Wageningen

The Netherlands

I. INTRODUCTION

The large polymeric molecules, cellulose, lignin, and hemicellulose, are the major components of plant cell walls. Taken in that order, they represent the three most abundant organic compounds on earth. Yet there are no known endogenous enzymes (as there are for starch or proteins) in the digestive system of vertebrates capable of converting them into smaller units that can be absorbed from the intestine. Digestion of the carbohydrates, cellulose, and hemicellulose, is by exogenous enzymes secreted by bacteria and protozoa living symbiotically in the gut of the animal. The absorbed end products are not the basic monomeric units of the molecule but volatile fatty acids, mainly acetic, propionic and butyric acids, with smaller amounts of branched-chain fatty acids. In ruminants, the site of this fermentation process is the rumen, which is an enlarged portion of the stomach. In monogastric herbivorous animals it occurs in a specially adapted cecum. Man and other monogastric nonherbivores do not have an extensively developed cecal fermentation system and are therefore incapable of digesting large amounts of vegetable fiber.

In contrast to the carbohydrate components of the plant cell wall, lignin is probably not attacked by intestinal enzymes of either endogenous or exogenous origin. Moreover, it hinders any breakdown of the cell wall carbohydrates by physically preventing access of the enzyme to its substrate, by forming an indigestible covalent linkage with the carbo-

hydrate, or by having a toxic effect on the micro-organisms
secreting the enzyme. As plants age, the proportion of
lignin increases and the digestibility of cellulose and hemicellulose declines. It is likely that the effect of lignin
on the digestibility of the cell-wall carbohydrates depends
on the part of the plant, its species or age, but this cannot be established until we have some idea of how the chemistry of lignin and its relationship to the cell-wall carbohydrates change with these factors.

Relative to grasses, legumes are characterized by small
amounts of hemicellulose and thus total cell wall. This
means that (1) the chemical and physical relationship
between lignin and the cell-wall carbohydrate in these two
groups of plants will be different, and (2) legumes will
have larger concentrations of soluble cell contents than
grasses at approximately similar stages of maturity. Legumes
will therefore have the greater digestibility, since the true
digestibility of the cell contents, which are independent of
the amount of lignin present, is almost 100% (97).

The effect of lignin on digestibility is shown in
Figure 1. The difference between grasses and legumes is
not as obvious as that found by Van Soest (96) who compared
the digestibility of dry matter rather than of organic matter with the lignin content.

In man the effect of lignin in depressing the digestibility of cellulose and hemicellulose is relatively unim-
portant, since these compounds are quantitatively minor
constituents of his diet. In recent years, however, dietary
lignin has been recognized as having a potentially beneficial
metabolic effect through its ability to combine with bile
salts secreted into the duodenum and prevent their subsequent
resorption in the large intestine. This interference in the
enterohepatic circulation of bile salts is thought to result
in a lowering of blood cholesterol levels. However, the
magnitude of the effect will depend on the chemical structure,
properties, and amount of lignin ingested.

This chapter reviews what is presently known of the
chemical structure of lignin and discusses common methods
of lignin analysis. Since most of the work has been done by
chemists working in the pulp and paper industry, much of the
information relates to lignin from trees; that which is avail-

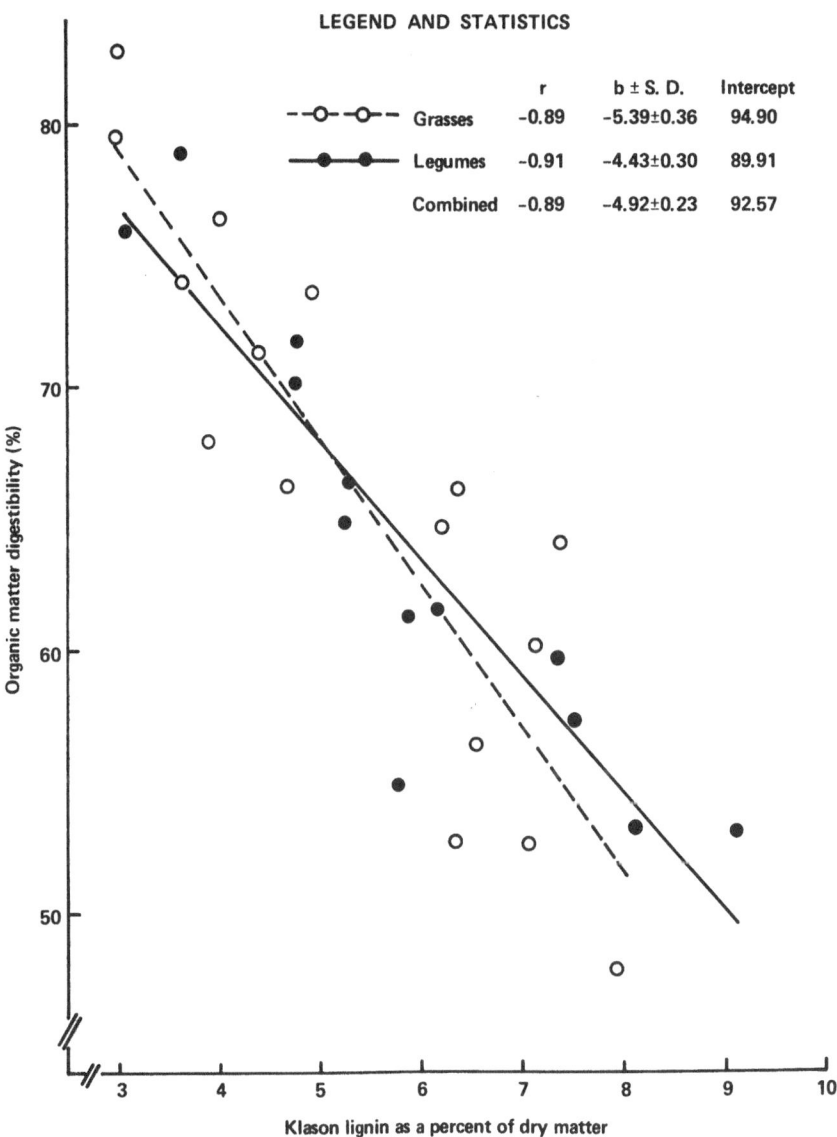

Figure 1. The relationship between the lignin content of grasses and legumes and the digestibility of their organic matter by sheep. From B. D. E. Gaillard. Calculation of the digestibility for ruminants of roughages from the contents of cell-wall constituents (69, 96).

able for lignins from herbaceous plants relates to work with
forage plants rather than with the vegetables and cereal
grains consumed by humans. Of the few papers that have
dealt with the lignin content of human foodstuffs, one (59)
is of little value because of inaccuracies in the method
used; the most recent[1] (98) gave analyses for only a select
few foods and was not a comprehensive survey.

II. STRUCTURE OF THE PLANT CELL WALL

In young, growing, undifferentiated plant cells, the
cytoplasm is surrounded by a primary cell wall, which consists mainly of cellulose fibrils embedded in a matrix of
pectin and hemicellulose and a unique hydroxyproline-rich
glycoprotein representing 2 to 10% of the plant cell wall
(93). As cell growth ceases, a secondary cell wall composed
of three distinct layers of cellulose microfibrils is laid
down between the cytoplasm and the primary cell wall. The
space between cell walls is occupied by the middle lamella.
Lignin is first deposited in the corners of the primary cell
wall, later extending into the middle lamella at the cell
corners. Lignification then spreads along the middle lamella into the secondary cell wall (101). When lignification
is complete, the highest concentration of lignin is found
in the middle lamella, but most of the total lignin (e.g.,
70%) is found in the secondary cell wall. Cells with unusually predominant secondary walls and large deposits of lignin are to be found in the vascular and supportive tissues
of plants. Coniferous wood (softwood) averages about 29%
lignin, 28% hemicellulose, and 43% cellulose, while wood
from broad-leafed trees (hardwood) contains about 22% lignin,
35% hemicellulose, and 43% cellulose (36). Nonwoody or herbaceous plants may contain between 0 and 25% lignin, depending on the age of the plant.

------

[1]Author's note: Since the preparation of this chapter, a more
recent publication dealing with the fiber and lignin contents
of human foodstuffs has appeared, namely that by A. A. McCon-
nell and M. A. Eastwood: A comparison of methods of measuring
"fibre" in vegetable material, J. Sci. Fd. Agric., 25:1451,
1974.

III. THE CHEMISTRY OF LIGNIN

A. Empirical Formulae

One of the earliest-discovered chemical features of lignin was the fact that it contains a high content of carbon (about 60%). This is because it is aromatic in nature; its building units are based on the substance hydroxyphenylpropane (I, Figure 2), which has a propane (C_3) sidechain attached to a benzene (C_6) ring. For this reason, the empirical formula of lignin is generally expressed on the basis of a C_9 unit (28). That for an average spruce (a softwood) lignin is $C_9H_{7.95}O_{2.4}(OCH_3)_{0.92}$ (28).

The alphabetic designation of the carbons in the sidechain for compounds II, III, and IV shown in Figure 2 follows the international nomenclature used by Freudenberg (28), but because many workers designate the benzyl carbon as $\propto$ and the terminal carbon as β, it is often less confusing to avoid this and use the terms, terminal, middle, and benzyl carbons.

B. Coupling of Lignin Monomers

The precise mechanism by which the individual monomers are linked has been discussed in a number of papers (11, 12, 13, 27, 37, 53, 81, 90).

It is proposed to summarize the subject so that the reader will, as Harkin (37) suggests, at least know the rules of the process even if he does not know the detailed constitution of say, spruce lignin. The structure of many of the compounds mentioned appears in Figure 2, and a summary of the nomenclature of the cinnamyl alcohols, aldehydes, and acids is given in Table 1, since these compounds are considered to be quantitatively the most important building blocks of lignins from trees.

When coniferyl alcohol (II) is incubated in the presence of air with a phenol oxidase enzyme (laccase) obtained from the juice of the mushroom Psalliota campestris (= Agaricus campestris), a cream-colored precipitate is formed which is chemically very similar to the lignin obtained from spruce

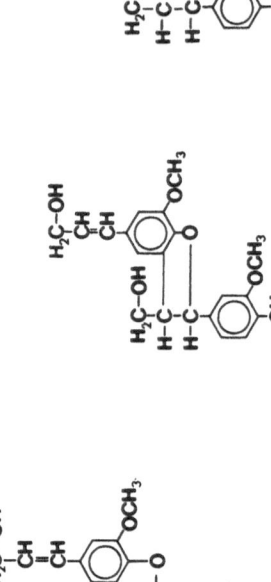

Figure 2a. Chemical structures of some lignin intermediates and model compounds.

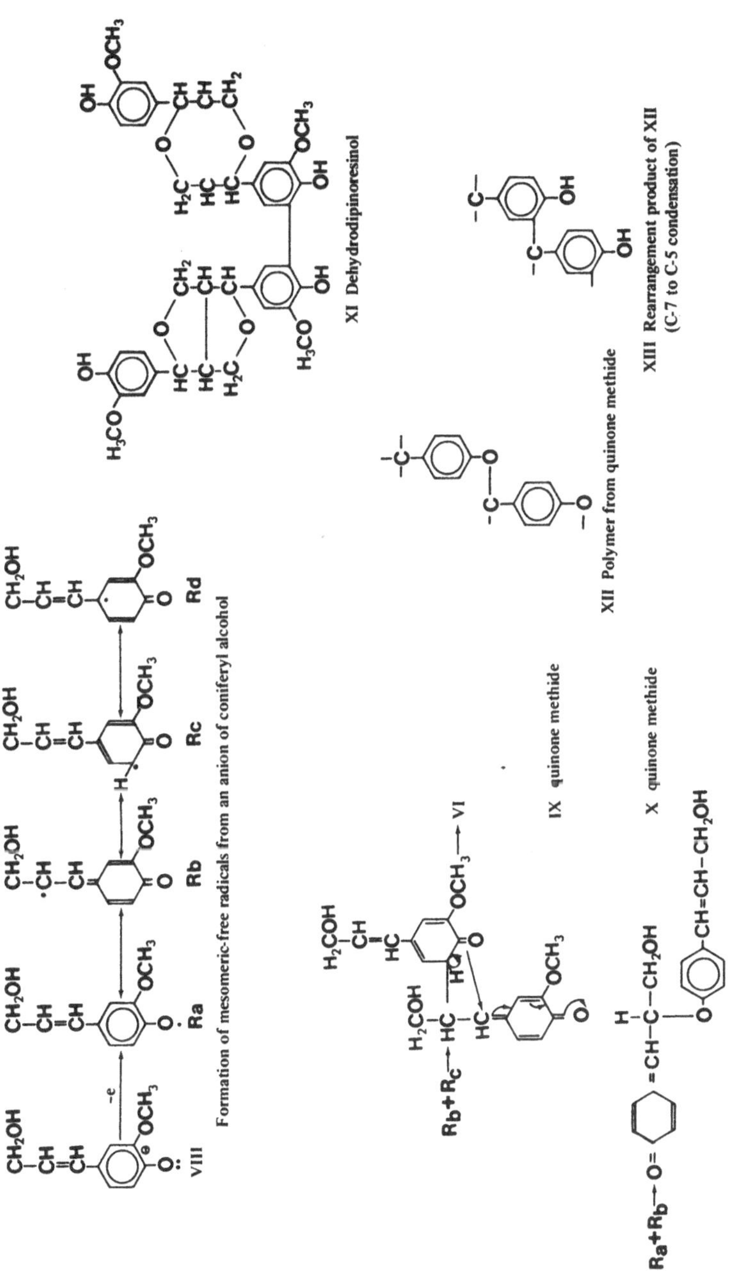

Figure 2b. Chemical structures of some lignin intermediates and model compounds.

TABLE 1. Derivatives of p-Hydroxycinnamyl Alcohols (Compounds II, III, IV)

Number of methoxyl groups in aromatic nucleus	0 p-Hydroxybenzyl nucleus	1 Guaiacyl nucleus	2 Syringyl nucleus
Alcohol Systematic Trivial	p-Hydroxycinnamyl p-Coumaryl	3-Methoxy-p-hydroxycinnamyl Coniferyl	3,5 Dimethoxy-p-hydroxycinnamyl Sinapyl
Aldehyde Systematic Trivial	p-Hydroxycinnam-aldehyde p-Coumaraldehyde	3-Methoxy-p-hydroxycinnam-aldehyde Coniferaldhyde	3,5 Dimethoxy-p-hydroxycinnam-aldehyde Sinapaldehyde
Acid Systematic Trivial	p-Hydroxycinnamic p-Coumaric	3-Methoxy-p-hydroxycinnamic Ferulic	3,5 Dimethoxy-p-hydroxycinnamic Sinapic
Products of alkaline nitrobenzene oxidation	p-Hydroxy-benzaldehyde	Vanillin	Syringaldehyde

wood. This artificial lignin was called dehydrogenation
polymer (DHP) by Karl Freudenberg, who was the first to
prepare it. p-Hydroxycinnamyl (coumaryl) alcohol (III)
likewise forms a dehydrogenation polymer (DHP-C), but
sinapyl alcohol (IV) alone, does not.

In fact, spruce lignin appears to be derived from
a mixture of 80% coniferyl alcohol, 14% p-coumaryl alcohol,
and 6% sinapyl alchol, since the DHP produced from such a
mixture has the same composition as the average spruce
lignin. Hardwood lignins appear to be derived from a cinnamyl alcohol mixture containing similar quantities of
coniferyl and sinapyl alcohol, with little p-coumaryl alcohol. Since the difference between these alcohols lies in
the number of methoxyl groups attached to the benzene ring,
the methoxyl content of the DHP or lignin produced from them
will reflect the composition of the original mixture dehydrogenated. Hardwood lignins, therefore, contain more methoxyl
groups than softwood lignins because a greater proportion
of sinapyl alcohol in the mixture is dehydrogenated. Dehydrogenation is not limited to mixtures of the three cinnamyl
alcohols; also it takes place in their higher oxidation
states, the aldehydes and acids that occur as intermediates
in the biosynthesis of the cinnamyl alcohols from phenyl-
alanine and, in grasses, tyrosine (68). This accounts for
the presence of aldehyde, carboxyl and lactone groups in
lignin. Pew and Connors (73) have shown that various
p-hydroxypropiophenones also undergo enzymic dehydrogenation,
which would also account for the presence of methyl, ethyl,
and aliphatic ester groups in lignins.

Intermediate products during the production of DHP from
coniferyl alcohol have been identified. Quantitatively, the
most significant dimers (dilignols) isolated are guaiglyc-
erol-β-coniferyl ether (V), dehydrodiconiferyl alcohol (VI),
and DL-pinoresinol (VII). To explain the formation of these
dilignols and other oligolignols that have either been found
in the DHP reaction mixture or been extracted from wood lignins with various solvents, Freudenberg (27) has proposed
the following mechanism.

It begins with the ionization of the phenolic hydroxyl
of the monomer (in this case coniferyl alcohol) to form the
anion (VIII) which, under the influence of the laccase enzyme,
loses an electron (in plants an enzyme, peroxidase, may have

the same function by transferring H to H_2O_2) to form the
free-radical R_a. The unpaired electron is distributed
throughout the molecule forming the free radicals R_b, R_c,
and R_d. Two R_b radicals can join through the middle carbons
of their sidechains, and if they are imagined to rotate about
this bond, the two dialkyl ether linkages of pinoresinol VII
can form. One estimate suggests that less than 12% of the
phenylpropanoid units in lignin have this type of linkage.
R_b and R_c can combine to form a transient dimeric quinone
methide (IX) linked by a -C-C- bond. Loss of a proton from
the upper quinone methide means that it is rearomatized and
a phenoxide ion (analagous to R_a) is formed. This ion then
shares its unpaired electron with the benzyl carbon of the
adjacent quinone methide, which is thereby also rearomatized,
and a new phenoxide ion is formed. This gains a proton to
form dehydrodiconiferyl alcohol (VI). Phenylcoumaran structures such as that found in dehydrodiconiferyl alcohol may
link about 20% of all the phenylpropanoid units in spruce
milled wood lignin (37).

The combination between R_a and R_b yields a dimeric p-
quinone methide (X), but the initial linkage is an alkyl
aryl ether link instead of a -C-C- link, and one ring is
already aromatic. The benzyl carbon in the quinone methide
(IX) is nucleophilically attacked by an ionic species formed
within the molecule itself (the phenoxide anion), but with
the other quinone methide (X), the nucleophilic attack can
come from an external nucleophile such as water, sugars or
other polysaccharides and probably the phenoxide anions of
other lignols. This causes the rearomatization of the
second ring, and the alkyl aryl ether is now an arylglycerol-β-aryl ether, which is the most common linkage of all in
spruce lignin, accounting for almost half of the cyclopro-
panoid units (37). If water is the attacking nucleophile,
then guaiacylglycerol-β-coniferyl ether (V) is formed. If
the nucleophile is the phenoxide anion of another lignol
(e.g., V, VI, VII or higher lignols), then trilignols or
oligolignols will result, and the molecule grows without
the necessity for further dehydrogenation. Finally, if
sugars or polysaccharides provide the nucleophile, it is
obvious that the lignin will be linked onto the polysaccharide. Both sorbitol and sucrose have been shown to give
benzyl alkyl ethers by this mechanism, and it is thought to
be the main mechanism whereby lignin is linked to polysaccharides.

Another frequently occurring link is the biaryl link, which may account for up to 25% of the interlignol units (37). An example is dehydrodipinoresinol (XI), which is a dimer of pinoresinol and is formed by the combination of two R_c-type units. The frequency of the biaryl link should be less in lignins that have a high proportion of syringyl units (e.g., hardwood lignins) and more in lignins with a preponderance of unmethoxylated nuclei (e.g., softwoods). Saturation of the sidechain prevents formation of the R_b-type radical, and thus oligolignols, whose sidechain must be more saturated than the monolignols, will be more prone to this type of linkage.

Diaryl ether bonds, formed by a combination of R_a- and R_c-type radicals, are also favored by saturation of the sidechain, but they account for only about 6% of the phenylpropanoid units in lignin (37).

A variety of other linkage structures have been isolated from wood lignins, and these are discussed in detail by Harkin (37). He states that the only coupling combination for which there is as yet no evidence are those between R_a and R_a, R_d and R_d and finally between R_c and R_d. Of these three, he considers only the first possibility unlikely. The last two possibilities may account for some of the products observed by Pew and Connors (73) upon enzymic dehydrogenation of proprioguaiacone.

As pointed out earlier, the lignin molecule can grow by the addition to quinone methides (IX) of phenols, which do not have to first be enzymatically dehydrogenated. This growth mechanism competes with another whereby the p-quinone methides themselves readily polymerize forming chains of noncyclic benzyl (C-γ)-aryl ethers (XII), which account for 10 to 12% of the phenylpropanoid units in spruce lignin (37). These may rearrange (C-γ to C-5 condensation) to form, in yet another growth mechanism, the structure shown in (XIII). Condensation of the C-γ can also occur, though to a lesser extent, with carbons number 6 or 2 of the adjacent ring (27).

In summary, there are four basic mechanisms of lignin polymerization, which are (1) repeated phenol dehydrogenation, (2) addition to quinone methides without further dehydrogenation, (3) polymerization of quinone methides to form noncyclic benzyl aryl ethers and (4) rearrangement of benzyl aryl ethers.

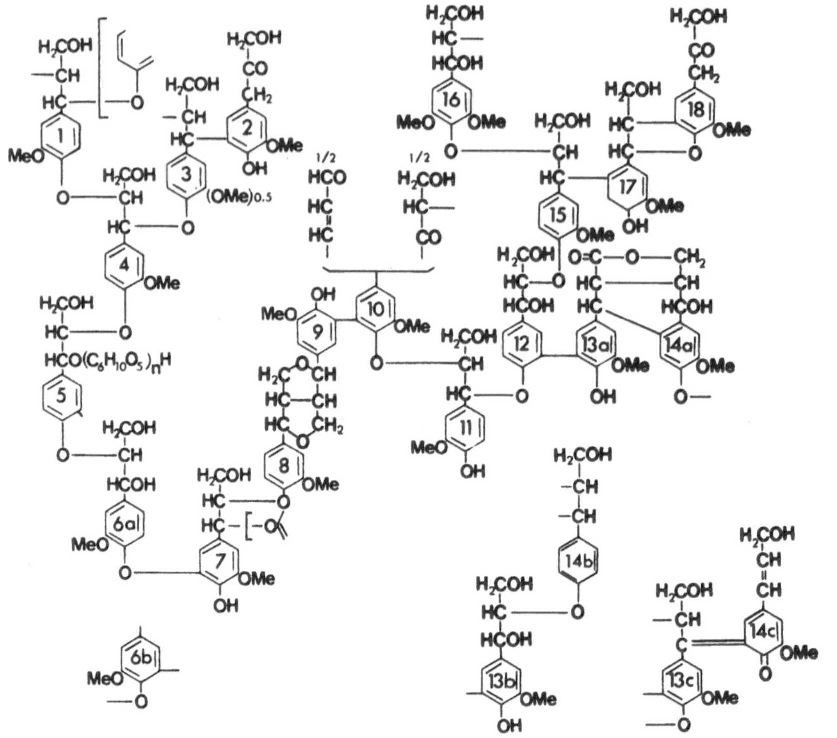

Figure 3.   Structure of spruce lignin according to
             Freudenberg.

A diagrammatic representation of spruce lignin as pic-
tured by Freudenberg (27) is given in Figure 3. Nimz (70)
has presented a scheme for the structure of beech lignin.

As is implied in the above discussion, the formation of
radical types R_a through R_d is not limited to those formed
from coniferyl alcohol; ferulic acid (85, 86: the acid analogue of coniferyl alcohol), coniferaldehyde (the aldehyde
analogue), p-coumaryl (III) and sinapyl (IV) alcohols and
their acid and aldehyde analogues and oligolignols themselves
can feasibly form all or some of the radicals analogous to
R_a through R_c. It has been shown, for example, that coniferyl alcohol can be enzymatically dehydrogenated to coniferaldehyde and further to <u>cis</u> and <u>trans</u> ferulic acid, and

these can be considered as genuine monolignols (37). Combination of the R_c analogue of coniferaldehyde with the R_b form of coniferyl alcohol yields, by a mechanism similar to the formation of dehydrodiconiferyl alcohol, an unsaturated aldehydic dilignol. This type of aldehyde structure represents about 3% of all the phenylpropanoid units in spruce lignin. Likewise a combination of an R_b analogue of trans ferulic acid with the coniferyl alcohol radical R_b forms a compound, pinoresinolide, which is similar to pinoresinol except that it has a lactone ring that contributes to the small lactone content (3 to 4%) of lignin. Ligninolide is similar to pinoresinolide in coming from ferulic acid and coniferyl alcohol, but only the lactone ring is formed, and the benzyl alkyl ether linkage does not occur because the middle carbon of the ferulic acid moiety loses a proton, forming a double bond with the benzyl carbon. Stafford (89) postulates that with grass lignins, a major portion is a polymer of ferulic acid and its oxidation products, while the rest is composed of a polymer of coniferyl aldehyde or its alcohol and their oxidation products associated with varying amounts of syringyl units. If this were so, one would expect a high concentration of lactone groups in grass lignins.

Sinapyl alcohol (IV) and its aldehyde and acid analogues have methoxyl groups at both the 3 and 5 positions of the benzene ring which prevent the formation of the R_a radical. Thus they are more limited in the number of ways they can combine with other mono- and oligolignols.

C. Structure of Lignins in Herbaceous Plants

Because of their suitability for radio tracer experiments, herbaceous plants, particularly grasses, have been used to establish the biochemical pathways leading to the formation of lignin monomers, but relatively little research has been directed at the structure per se of the lignin in such plants. It is assumed that the various types of lignin linkages which occur in woody plants also occur in herbaceous plants. It is therefore of interest to review the work that has been done relating to the structure of herbaceous lignins, since it is these, mainly in the form of vegetables and cereal grain, which are likely to be consumed by humans.

Ester Linkages in Grasses. While wood lignins appeared
to be derived by dehydrogenation of either coniferyl alcohol
(softwoods) or a mixture of coniferyl and sinapyl alcohols
(hardwoods), grass lignins appeared to be derived from a
mixture of the above alcohols with a significant proportion
of p-coumaryl alcohol, because on alkaline nitrobenzene oxidation, considerable amounts of p-hydroxybenzaldehyde were
obtained, in addition to vanillin and syringaldehyde (18).
See Table 1. Kuć and Nelson (49), Gee et al. (29), and
Kuć et al. (50) found that significant amounts of p-coumaric
acid (e.g., 5 to 13% of the total lignin) in corn plants
were esterified to the rest of the lignin molecule, which
they termed the lignin core. This acid would yield p-hydroxybenzaldehyde on alkaline nitrobenzene oxidation. Moreover,
four mutant genes, which affect the amount and type of lignin
in corn, reduced the amount of p-coumaric acid so esterified
(50). Smaller amounts of ferulic acid (e.g., 3 to 9% of the
total lignin) were likewise esterified, but the amount was
less affected by the presence of a single mutant gene and
increased by the presence of two.

Gee et al. (29) suggested that p-coumaric acid may be
doubly esterified (i.e., at both its carboxyl and phenolic
hydroxyl ends), linking two lignin cores, while ferulic acid
is part of a polymerizing core prior to appreciable cross
linking. Prior to this work, Stafford (88) had detected
large amounts of p-coumaric and ferulic acids in alkaline
extracts from Phleum pratense. She suggested that the acids
may have been products of ester linkages. Higuchi et al.
(41, 42) firmly established the presence of ester linkages
between the core lignin of grasses and p-coumaric and ferulic
acids. In milled wood lignin (MWL) preparations from seven
grass species, esterified ferulic acid constituted between
0.1 and 0.6% and p-coumaric acid constituted between 2.6 and
9.8% of the lignin preparations (42). In MWL from three non-
grass monocotyledons, there were only traces of ferulic acid,
while p-coumaric acid ranged from trace amounts in Smilax
china to 0.3% in Asparagus officinalis. Shimada (83) concluded that the majority of p-coumaric acid in bamboo and
grass lignins are linked through their carboxyl group with
a hydroxyl group on the terminal carbon of the core lignin
sidechain. Shimada (83) has suggested that in the plant,
the p-coumaryl group is enzymatically transferred to the
lignin core. Miksche (64) has pointed out that cinnamic
acids may be incorporated into wheat lignin by ways other

than esterification. This is in accord with Stafford's (89)
postulate that grass lignins are partly composed of polymers
of ferulic acid.

Ester linkages of ferulic and p-coumaric acids may not
be restricted to linkages with the lignin core. El-Basyouni
and Towers (24) extracted wheat plants with ethanol, which
removed ethanol-soluble esters of a number of phenolic acids
including ferulic and p-coumaric acids. Cold alkaline hydrolysis of the ethanol-insoluble residue released three
phenolic compounds, two of which were ferulic and p-coumaric
acids. These cell-wall-bound or ethanol-insoluble esters
were considered to be intermediates in lignin biosynthesis,
although undoubtedly much of the acids was derived from the
lignin core. Hartley (40) found that a carbohydrate-ferulic
acid ester is released from the cell walls of Lolium multiflorum by digestion with a cellulase enzyme. It is unknown
what proportion of the cinnamic acid esters in the cell wall
are involved in links with lignin and nonlignin fractions.

Other Chemical and Physical Properties. It has been
shown by several workers (74, 77, 79, 91) that the methoxyl
content of lignin increases with the age of the plant, which
means that there is an increase in the proportion of methoxy-
lated units, especially sinapyl units, in the mixture being
dehydrogenated to form lignin. Stone et al. (91) showed
that the increase in methoxyl content was accompanied by an
increase in the proportion of syringaldehyde and, to a lesser
extent, in the proportion of vanillin obtained upon alkaline
nitrobenzene oxidation of wheat plant lignins. Even within
one plant the methoxyl content of the lignin can differ, as
shown by analyses of lignin from peanut (Arachis hypogaea L.)
pod shell (6.5% methoxyl), root (10.0%), stem (8.4%), and
foliage (2.9%) (82). The inhomogeneity of lignin within one
plant and even one cell has been emphasized by Miksche (64)
and Stafford (88).

Bondi and Meyer (7) found a striking difference between
grasses and legumes in the methoxyl content of their alkali
lignins. Alkali lignins from bersem clover (Trifolium alexandrinum bersem) contained 5.1% methoxyl groups, fahli clover
(T. alexandrinum fahli), 5.8%, and peanut hay (Arachis hypogaea), 4.3%; while Eragrostis tef contained 9.6%, Pencillaria
sp., 9.7%, and Setaria italica, 9.6% methoxyl. Methylation
with diazomethane (which substitutes methoxyl groups for aro-

matic hydroxyl groups) trebled the methoxyl content of the
legume alkali lignins but only doubled that of the grasses,
which suggested that the excess methoxyl groups in the
grasses corresponded to unsubstituted hydroxyl groups in
the lucerne. Gordon (32) confirmed these results using
alkali lignins prepared according to processes used by Bondi
and Meyer (7) from alfalfa (Medicago sativa) and a mixture
of grasses composed mainly of Bromus inermis. The legume
alkali lignin contained 7.9% methoxyl and that of the grass
mixture, 11.9% when expressed on an amino-acid-free basis.
A negative reaction to anthrone suggested carbohydrates were
absent from the preparations. However, the corresponding
Klason lignins (corrected for Nx6.25) contained 12.6% and
13.0% methoxyl, respectively. With legumes, either alkali
extracts a specific fraction of lignin, which is low in
methoxyl groups, or it extracts much nonproteinaceous and
noncarbohydrate material with the lignin. The alkali lignins
from the alfalfa had more carbon (61.9%) than the grass lignin (60.3%), which attests to the aromatic nature of the
preparation and supports the former possibility.

Legume lignins are much less soluble in alkali than
grass lignins (32, 65, 96). For example, Gordon (32) extracted only about 30% of alfalfa lignin with alkali compared with about 60% for grass lignin. Reaction of the
plant material with thioglycolic acid (See Section IV-B
below) gives higher yields of lignin, but it is combined
with thioglycolic acid. The lignin in this lignothioglycolic
acid product is, according to Freudenberg (28), probably
closer in structure to the original lignin than any other
lignin preparation except milled-wood lignin (MWL, IV-B
below). A comparison of the composition of the alkali lignins and lignin from the lignothioglycolic acids (before
correcting for the presence of thioglycolic acid as described
by Freudenberg (28) from the grass and lucerne referred to
above is given in Table 2. The composition of MWL prepared
from these plants as described by Freudenberg (28) is given
in Table 3. There were considerable amounts of carbohydrate
present in the MWL, which accounts for their low content of
carbon and methoxyl groups.

Although alfalfa alkali lignins contained more total
hydrogen (protons) than the grass, they contained only two
thirds as many aromatic protons. This suggested they were
more highly cross-linked lignins (32). Further evidence of
this was the fact that they also had fewer uncondensed p-hy-

TABLE 2. Composition of Various Lignin Preparations
From a Mixed Grass Hay and an Alfalfa Hay
and the Feces of Sheep Consuming These Hays

	Elements				$-OCH_3$
	C	H	N	S	
Grass					
Feed Klason[1]	56.3	6.5	1.5	2.1	11.1
Feed Klason[2]	56.8	7.0	1.5	3.2	13.6
Feces Klason[1]	59.0	6.7	1.7		11.8
Feces Klason[2]	57.1	7.3	1.6		12.5
Feed alkali[3]	63.2	6.3	1.3		12.1
Feces alkali[3]	61.1	6.3	1.1		11.6
Feed LTHA[4]	53.8	5.5	2.0	7.3	
Feces LTHA[4]	54.9	5.5	1.6	7.6	10.4
Alfalfa					
Feed Klason[1]	59.5	6.5	1.7	2.0	10.5
Feed Klason[2]	57.9	7.3	2.0	2.7	11.4
Feces Klason[1]	59.6	7.0	2.1		11.6
Feces Klason[2]	58.3	7.2	1.1		11.6
Feed alkali[3]	64.3	7.4	2.9		7.5
Feces alkali[3]	64.1	7.2	1.9		8.1
Feed LTHA[4]	56.1	6.1	2.4	6.9	
Feces LTHA[4]	54.3	5.6	1.7	8.4	11.7

[1]Method of Ellis et al. (25)
[2]Method of Van Soest (94). Klason lignins are on an ash-
  free basis.
[3]Corrected for contributions from amino acids.
[4]LTHA, lignothioglycolic acids.

TABLE 3. Composition of Lignin–Carbohydrate Complexes Extracted From
Ball–milled Forages with Dioxane:Water (9:1)

Forage	Yield (% K.L.)[1]	Elements					Total (%)	Carbohydrate Ratios (%)				
		C	H	N	S	-OCH$_3$		Gal[2]	Gluc[2]	Ara[2]	Xyl[2]	Rha[2]
Mixed grass hay	6.8	55.5	6.3	1.8	1.1	3.9	35.5	5.5	44.1	17.7	16.4	16.4
Alfalfa hay	15.0	54.0	0.7	0.9	0.8	7.3	25.4	12.1	40.9	15.9	23.5	7.6
Troyer Reid maize	22.7	57.5	5.5	0.8	0.8	9.9	18.9	3.9	18.1	7.5	70.6	0.0
Brown mid-rib maize	29.5	54.3	5.4	0.9	0.9	9.3	11.5	0.0	28.2	9.2	62.6	0.0

See p. 52 of reference 28 for description of method; also from unpublished work by Gordon.

[1] K.L., Klason lignin by method of Ellis et al. (25). The low yield for the grass hay is due to the fact that it was extracted for only 12 hours with the dioxane:water, whereas the other three samples were extracted for 72 hours.

[2] Gal, galactose; Gluc, glucose; Ara, arabinose; Xyl, xylose; Rha, rhamnose.

droxybenzyl alcohol groups than the lignin grass. On the
other hand, they had a much greater proportion of protons
on the sidechain which were probably due to methyl groups,
perhaps arising from the dehydrogenation of propriophenones
(73).

Moon and Abou-Raya (65) found that the lignin remaining
after alkali extraction of plant (grasses and legumes) and
fecal material could be removed by ethylacetoacetate. This
lignin was much less contaminated with protein and had a
higher methoxyl content than the lignin previously removed
with alkali, even when a correction was made for the amount
of protein present. They attributed the difference to contamination (carbohydrate?), but part of it could have reflected a real difference in the type of lignin extracted by alkali and acetoacetate, particularly with the legumes.

Lignin-Carbohydrate Linkages. A mechanism for the possible formation of covalent links between lignin and carbohydrate was described earlier. The evidence for the presence
of such linkages was reviewed by Merewether (62) in 1957.
A more recent review is that of Lai and Sarkanen (52). Certainly some and perhaps most of the lignin in woody and
herbaceous plants is covalently linked to carbohydrate
(probably mainly hemicellulose), but the exact nature of
the bonding has not been identified as yet. In ryegrass,
Morrison (67) has postulated that at least three types of
bonding may be present, namely one cleaved on borohydride
reduction, another cleaved by alkali, and a linkage resistant to alkali. Gordon (32) has isolated alkali-stable lignin-
carbohydrate complexes from feed and feces of sheep consuming
Zea mays, a mixed grass hay, and Medicago sativa. There is
probably a whole range of lignin-carbohydrate complexes in
any one plant which differ in their proportions of lignin
and carbohydrate and the nature of the linkages involved.
Differences in the natures of such complexes are going to
play a major role in the effects of ingested lignin during
digestion. Bjorkman (5) and Brownell (15) have described
"standardized" solvent extraction procedures for isolating
lignin-carbohydrate complexes from milled wood.

The composition of some lignin-carbohydrate complexes
extracted from some forage plants is given in Table 3.

D.   Chemical Reactivity of Some Interlignol Links

A knowledge of the stability of the chemical linkages
in lignin is important in deciding what procedure to use
for extracting lignin from plant tissues or for determining
the total amount of lignin in the plant, and also in evaluating possible changes that may occur to lignin as a result of
passage through the digestive tract. Table 4 summarizes the
various types of linkages which have been found in a variety
of lignins from various sources. In general, -C-C- bonds
are much more stable to both acid and alkali than ether bonds,
and benzyl-0-4 and β-0-4 links are susceptible to hydrolysis
by acids and bases, while most other bonds in lignin are
largely unhydrolyzable.

The two most important factors that govern the effect
of chemical agents on lignin are the type of functional
group at the benzyl carbon and the presence of free phenolic
hydroxyl groups. Acid hydrolysis of lignin causes the benzyl
alcohols to form carbonium ions (R_3C^+), which in strongly
acid solutions condense onto an aromatic nucleus. This
results in a decrease in the solubility of the lignin and
often its precipitation from solution. Lignin is quite
soluble in alkali, but on alkaline hydrolysis, condensation
reactions can still occur because of the formation of quinone
methides from units containing free hydroxyl groups. Etheri-
fication of both benzyl and phenolic hydroxyl groups therefore render other lignin linkages more stable. Provided the
phenolic hydroxyl group is free, the number of uncondensed
p-hydroxybenzyl alcohol groups can be estimated by reacting
with quinone monochloroimide, which yields a blue dyestuff
with such compounds (30). p-Hydroxybenzyl alcohols with an
0,0'-dihydroxybiphenyl linkage do not react positively in
this test (73). The frequency of the free phenolic hydroxyl
groups can be determined spectrophotometrically (3, 31, 102;
also see section IV-B below).

The weakest interlignol links in lignin are the noncyclic benzyl aryl ethers, which are readily hydrolyzed by
both acids and alkali, and even lukewarm water provided
p-hydroxyl substituents are present (53). Hardwoods have
more of such bonds than softwoods.

Phenylcoumaran structures with a free phenolic group
are readily broken down in hot alkali by fracture of the

TABLE 4.   Classification of Types of Chemical Links in
Lignin and Their Frequency

---

1.   Ethers

1.1   Benzyl (γ) ethers

1.1.1   Cyclic

1.1.1.1   Benzyl alkyl ethers, e.g., in pinoresinol
          (10 to 12%)

1.1.1.2   Benzyl aryl ethers, phenylcoumaran structure (20%)

1.1.2   Noncyclic (>12%)

1.1.2.1   Benzyl alkyl ethers, e.g., lignin-polysaccharide

1.1.2.2   Benzyl (γ) aryl ethers, formed by addition of
          phenols to quinone methides or polymerization
          of quinone methides themselves (10 to 12%; 15%)

1.2   Alkyl aryl ethers

1.2.1   Arylglycerol β aryl ether (β-0-4 alkyl aryl
          ethers) (<50%)

1.2.2   Methyl aryl ether (methoxyl groups)

1.3   Diaryl (biphenyl) ethers (6%), e.g., dehydro-
          dipinoresinol

2.   Lactones (3 to 4%)

2.1   Pinoresinolide type structure

2.2   Lignenolide type structure

3.   Ester bonds

3.1   Linking noncore lignin

3.2   Linking aliphatic groups

3.3   Linking polysaccharides

4.   C-C bonds

4.1   Biaryl (25%)

4.2   Dialkyl, e.g., in pinoresinol

4.3   Aryl alkyl, e.g., in phenylcoumaran structure

benzyl aryl ether bond, although the -C-C- bond remains intact. Pinoresinol is also degraded by alkali if free phenolic groups are present. Provided the benzyl and/or terminal
carbons adjacent to the middle carbon contain free-OH groups
or the benzyl carbon has a carbonyl group, even nonphenolic
β-ether bonds are hydrolyzed by alkali, and since there is
no simultaneous formation of -C-C- bonds, extensive depoly-
merization can occur. These bonds are the most numerous of
all, at least in spruce lignin. The various ester bonds in
lignin will undergo saponification with alkali at room
temperature. This is more important in the case of grass
lignins where substantial amounts of p-hydroxycinnamic acids
(noncore lignin) are esterified to the rest of the lignin
molecule and can be released as the free acid by alkaline
hydrolysis. Methoxyl groups are generally resistant to
alkaline hydrolysis unless the temperature is raised to
around 200°C. Cleavage by hot alkali between the -C-C-
bonds of the sidechain of phenylpropanoid units can occur,
but quantitatively these reactions are probably not very
important.

Hydrolysis with acid cleaves a variety of ether linkages, but they are simultaneously replaced by -C-C- bonds
forming a more insoluble, highly condensed compound with an
increased carbon and reduced hydrogen content. However, on
hydrolysis with approximately 3% HCl in ethanol (ethanolysis),
most of the lignin is dissolved forming water soluble phenylpropanoid ketones called "Hibbert's ketones." Likewise much
lignin is dissolved, and some of these ketones and other
monomeric products are obtained if the lignin is refluxed
with 0.2 M HCl in dioxane:water (9:1). This process is
called "acidolysis." The ketones are considered to be derived
by cleavage of glycerol β-ether units. On hydrolysis of lignin with stronger concentrations of aqueous acid such as 12%
HCl or 29% H_2SO_4, as much as 4% formaldehyde has been obtained (10). It is formed from those units which contain a terminal methylol group and substituted in the benzyl or middle
carbons with hydroxyl or ether groups. The middle carbon
may contain, alternatively, an aryl group. Methoxyl groups
are split from lignin by hot concentrated H_2SO_4 forming
methanol. This is the basis of one method of determining
the methoxyl groups in lignin (61).

IV. ANALYTICAL METHODS FOR LIGNIN

A. Quantitative Determination

Because of the large variations in the chemical composition of lignin (e.g., the ratio of core to noncore lignin;
the frequency of certain linkage types, some of which are
more susceptible to chemical hydrolysis than others) and the
presence in highly variable amounts of other polyphenolic
(e.g., lignins, flavonoids) and nonpolyphenolic compounds
(carbohydrates, proteins) which may cocondense with lignin
either in vivo during plant growth or during the process of
lignin isolation or intestinal digestion, it is unlikely that
only one method of lignin determination will be applicable
for all species and ages of plants, or even for different
parts of the same plant or for the same plant before or
after digestion. The best method will be one that combines
general applicability with ease of analysis, although with
specific samples, modifications may be necessary.

Fischer (26) has reviewed the various methods used for
lignin analysis and their application to plant crops and
feedstuffs. This paper suggests that little improvement can
be made on the method of Ellis, Matrone, and Maynard (25),
a method which incorporated the basic principles of lignin
analysis established up until that time. The five essential
steps in this method are:

1. Removal of waxes, fats, and pigments
    (extraction)[1]

2. Removal of protein (proteolysis)[1]

3. Removal of hemicelluloses (prehydrolysis)[1]

4. Removal of cellulose (main hydrolysis)

5. Supplementing Step 4 and coagulation of
    any lignin dissolved in Step 4 (final
    hydrolysis).

Extraction is usually done with ethanol-benzene, proteolysis by digestion with 1% pepsin in 0.1 N HCl, prehydrolysis with 1 N (5%) H_2SO_4, main hydrolysis with 72% H_2SO_4, and
final hydrolysis with 0.6 N H_2SO_4 (3%). Klason lignin is

---
[1]Steps 1, 2, and 3 are called pretreatments.

defined in this chapter as any lignin isolated using strong
H_2SO_4 (usually 72%) to dissolve cellulose in the main hydrolysis step. Therefore, the lignin isolated by the method of
Ellis et al. (25) is a Klason lignin.

In 1963, Van Soest (95) introduced a method whereby a
Klason lignin is isolated using one pretreatment. Refluxing
with a detergent solution (2% cetyltrimethylammonium bromide)
in 1 N H_2SO_4 permits Steps 1, 2, and 3 to be done simultaneously, leaving a residue of acid-detergent fiber (ADF)
which is then subjected to the main hydrolysis. This, plus
the elimination of Step 5, means that the lignin determination can be done in a matter of hours rather than days.
Consequently, this method of lignin determination (acid-
detergent lignin, ADL) has become very popular.

The ADL method usually gives lower values than the
method of Ellis et al. (25), and with certain plants this
is due to a loss of lignin dissolved in the acid-detergent
solution (34, 76). For example, in a variety of Zea mays,
Gordon and Neudoerffer (34) obtained greater yields of alkali lignin than ADL. On the other hand, Donnelly and Wear
(22) concluded that tannin was present as a contaminant in
the Klason lignin from sericea lespedeza (Lespedeza cuneata)
when the method of Ellis et al. (25) was used but not when
the ADL method was used. Despite attempts to remove protein,
nitrogen is still a contaminant of the Klason lignins prepared by either method. The composition of Klason lignins
prepared by both methods appears in Table 2, where it can
be seen that the methods are about equally effective in removing protein. Most of the sulfur present presumably arises
from the sulfuric acid.

Hydrolyzing cell walls, prepared by using a neutral,
3% sodium lauryl sulfate solution (99) with 1.0 to 1.5
N H_2SO_4, removes hemicellulose; if this residue is subjected
to the main hydrolysis, the resultant Klason lignin has less
nitrogen and ash than ADL prepared from the same material
(unpublished work by the author).

It is important when using the method of Ellis et al.
that proteolysis precedes prehydrolysis, or the efficiency
of proteolysis is reduced and the subsequent Klason lignin
will have an increased nitrogen content. Thomas and Arm-

strong (94) consider that a correction should be made for the
content of crude protein (Nx6.25) present in the Klason lignin.

Another precaution that must be taken is to ensure that
the sample being analyzed has not been dried at temperatures
above 60°C. This subject was reviewed by Fischer (26). High
initial drying temperatures increase the apparent lignin
yield, especially with succulent or immature tissue and with
feces. At the present time most samples are freeze-dried
before analysis, and the production of artifact lignin from
excessive drying temperatures should not be a problem.

Apart from considerable alteration in the lignin structure, an important drawback in the Klason lignin procedure
is that variable amounts of lignin are soluble in 72% H_2SO_4
(58). Van Soest and Wine (100) introduced an alternative
to the ADL method whereby the ADF was treated with potassium
permanganate to remove the lignin and leave cellulose. This
method gave lignin values that were about 20% higher than
the ADL method. Cutin, which may be a significant contaminant of Klason lignins in seed hulls, is excluded in this
procedure. Instead of using permanganate, Edwards (23)
removed the lignin from ADF using triethylene glycol containing 0.2% HCl. This gave similar results to the permanganate method.

Many other methods of lignin determination have only
historical interest although some, such as that of Morrison
(66), may be suitable for routine determinations on relatively uniform materials. He adapted the spectral procedure
of Johnson, Moore, and Zank (45) to forages. Plant cell
walls are digested in a mixture of acetyl bromide and acetic
acid, and the ultraviolet absorbance has to be calibrated
against samples whose lignin content is determined by a Klason
procedure. It is probably better to determine the Klason lignin content directly if absolute rather than relative values
are required.

In conclusion, although all methods of lignin determination are arbitrary, probably the best general method available for estimating the total lignin content is a Klason
procedure based on that of Ellis et al. (25). The ADL procedure of Van Soest is simpler and faster, but at times it
underestimates the total lignin content.

B.   Qualitative Analysis

Because the Klason lignins are highly altered as a
result of treatment with strong acid, they are of little
use for chemical studies on the lignin. In general, the
higher the yield of lignin obtained, the greater is the
degree of its chemical alteration. On the other hand, extraction of a relatively unaltered lignin is associated with
yields which are so low that the product may not be representative of the total lignin. One alternative is to examine
the lignin in situ through, for example, the use of staining
techniques, ultraviolet and infrared light, and electron
microscopy (51). Two important staining techniques used
for studying the distribution of lignin in situ are the
Wiesner and Maüle reactions (51). In the Wiesner reaction,
a mixture of phloroglucinol and hydrochloric acid give a red
color in the presence of coniferaldehyde groups in lignin and
a blue color in the presence of sinapyl aldehyde. Vanillin
and syringaldehyde give a peach color. Although the reaction
has been widely used to demonstrate the presence of lignin,
certain chemical treatments that remove aldehyde groups result in a negative reaction even though lignin is present.
Thus, the intensity of the color is not a measure of the
degree of lignification.

For the Maüle reaction, the material is treated succes-
sively with dilute potassium permanganate, hydrochloric acid
and ammonium hydroxide. Angiosperm lignins stain a rose red
because of the presence of syringyl groups, while gymnosperm
lignins containing relatively few such components show only
a brownish color. Safranin-fast green staining is also used
but is less specific for lignin. Lignified cells stain red
with safranin, and fast green stains lignin-free tissues
green.

Purified lignins or lignins in situ can be degraded by
a variety of techniques to yield monomeric products that
give some idea of the constitution of the original lignin.
One method is the technique of alkaline nitrobenzene oxidation. As shown in Table 1, this process results in the formation of the three aldehydes, p-hydroxybenzaldehyde, vanillin,
and syringaldehyde. Various nonlignin phenolic compounds may
give rise to these products, so care should be taken to remove them first without removing any lignin. With grasses,
the p-coumaric and ferulic acids (noncore lignin) esterified

to the lignin core will give these products, although they
do not reflect the basic structure of the core lignin.
The procedure also results in the loss of the C_9-C_3 structure. Finally, the syringyl components of the lignin give
relatively more syringaldehyde than guaiacyl structures
give vanillin or p-hydroxybenzyl structures give p-hydroxybenzaldehyde. This is due to the fact that methoxyl groups
in the aromatic nucleus prevent intramolecular condensation
occurring. Thus p-coumaryl units are more condensed than
guaiacyl units, while syringyl units are the least condensed (28). Despite the above criticisms, alkaline nitrobenzene oxidation is a very common analytical tool, and a
number of papers (8, 21, 38, 72, 91) describe procedures for
the oxidation of whole-plant material and isolated lignins
and for separation of the products by gas-liquid chromatography. Other oxidative techniques of lignin degradation
have been discussed by Chang and Allan (16).

    A nonoxidative degradative procedure that retains the
C_6-C_3 structure of lignin in the monomeric products is that
called "ethanolysis," whereby plant material or purified
lignins are refluxed with ethanolic HCl (e.g., 2 g HCl/100
ml ethanol). Water-soluble phenylpropanoid ketones (Hibbert's ketones) are formed from arylglycerol-β-ether structures in which the aryl group is either an uncondensed unit
with a free phenolic hydroxyl group or is linked through
hydrolyzable benzyl-0-4 or β-0-4 bonds with the rest of the
lignin (52). Higuchi and Kawamura (43) used gas chromatography to fractionate ethanolysis products obtained from a
number of woody and nonwoody plants.

    The solubility of lignin in dioxane is increased by the
presence of both an acid catalyst (e.g., 0.5 to 0.2% HCl)
and up to 10% water (48). Refluxing plant material with such
a mixture (e.g., dioxane:water, 9:1 containing 0.2 N HCl)
results in considerable extraction of lignin which has not
undergone significant condensation changes. Simultaneously,
a variety of "acidolysis" monomers are produced, the major
ones being, at least in bamboo lignin, β-oxysinapyl alcohol
and its derivatives and β-oxyconiferyl alcohol and its derivatives (44). The separation and measurement of these
compounds by gas-liquid chromatography from MWL of bamboo,
beech, and Japanese red pine have been described by Higuchi
et al. (44).

It is also desirable to conduct studies on purified
lignin preparations, and a variety of extraction techniques
have been developed. The subject has been reviewed by Lai
and Sarkanen (52). The method thought to cause least changes
to the lignin is that of Bjorkman (4, 5), and the preparation
is called milled wood lignin (MWL). Yields of up to 50% of
the total Klason lignin have been obtained. The procedure
involves ball-milling the pre-extracted material in toluene
for a number of days, removal of the toluene and extraction
of the milled material with dioxane-water to remove the lignin. After evaporation of the dioxane-water, the crude lignin is dissolved in 90% acetic acid and precipitated into
water. It is further purified by dissolving in a 1,2 di-
chlorethane-ethanol mixture (2:1) and precipitated into
diethyl ether. The MWL usually contains 1 to 2% carbohydrate.

A simpler method for purifying the MWL has been described by Freudenberg (28) but, at least with herbaceous
plants, carbohydrate is still present (see Table 3).
Brownell (14, 15) has also reported a number of modifications to the procedure, including the elimination of the
need to use toluene as a grinding medium, the substitution
of a conventional ball mill for a vibratory mill and extraction of the lignin with a mixture of water, sodium thio-
cyanate, benzyl alcohol and dimethylformamide.

The lignin partions into the benzyl alcohol while lignin-carbohydrate complexes remain in the aqueous phase.
The dimethylformamide (1 to 2%) prevents emulsification but
increases the proportion of lignin-carbohydrate complexes
contaminating the organic phase.

A method that gives high yields of lignin is to react
the plant material with thioglycolic acid in 2 N HCl (52).
A solid lignothioglycolic acid is formed which can be isolated by alkaline hydrolysis of the links to other cell wall
components. The thioglycolic acids react with benzylhydroxyl
groups and phenylcoumaran structures. The content of sulfur
is measured (it is usually around 7 to 10%) and from this the
true lignin content of the complex is calculated as described
by Freudenberg (28). It is claimed (28, 52) that the lignothioglycolic acid is closer in structure to the original
lignin than any other lignin preparation except MWL. However, it can be seen in Table 2 that nitrogen contamination
is still a problem.

A lignin preparation that has been recommended (52) for studying grass lignins because of high yields and unaltered chemical structure is the alkali lignin. The lignin is extracted with alkali (e.g., 0.5 to 1.0 N NaOH or 10% KOH) at room temperature or with heating and the alkali extract acidified to precipitate a lignin-hemicellulose complex. Gordon (32) found that refluxing plant material for 6 hr with 10% KOH (49) resulted in alkali lignins with abnormal NMR spectra, so excessive heating should be avoided. The hemicellulose can be separated by adding ethanol to the alkaline extract prior to acidification (7), which causes the carbohydrate to precipitate. Repeated redissolving of the complex in alkali and reacidification has been claimed to result in a lignin containing no carbohydrate (49).

A major problem with lignin preparations from herbaceous plants is contamination with nitrogen. Although Freudenberg's picture of lignin structure in spruce has no place for nitrogen, Bondi and Meyer (7) regarded N as being an integral part of herbaceous lignins. Most workers, however, consider their preparations were contaminated with protein, although Meyer and Bondi (63) could detect no amino acids in the hydrolysates of alkali lignins. Whitehead and Quick (103) found that nitrogen in acidolysis lignins from grasses was present in the form of $-NCH_3$ groups. Gee, Nelson, and Kuć (29) used a relatively mild but low-yielding procedure to extract lignins from normal and bm_1 corns with dimethylformamide. These lignins all contained nitrogen, but they gave negative biuret tests for protein and negative colorimetric tests for indole groups; no amino acids were detected in alkaline hydrolysates of the lignins. Even MWL prepared from grasses by Higuchi and Kawamura (43) contained 0.3 to 0.4% N. Finally, work by the author (32, 34) has shown that while amino acids do contaminate alkali lignins, not all the nitrogen present can be accounted for as amino acids. It seems likely, therefore, that tertiary nitrogen can be present in lignin preparations, but whether it is incorporated through biosynthetic processes in the plant or is an artifact of the isolation procedure is the unanswered question. It is possible that nitrogenous compounds with free phenolic hydroxyl groups are incorporated by dehydrogenation into the lignin. However, Stafford (88) found that tyrosine, when incubated with Phleum pratense lamina in the presence of H_2O_2, failed to produce lignin-like polymers. Pepper and Wood (71) are apparently the only workers to report the isolation of lignin preparations with no nitro-

gen, but they make no comment on its absence. Their analysis
for oat straw acidolysis lignin was 69.26% C, 5.71% H, and
nil% N.

An important feature of any isolated lignin is its content of methoxyl groups. If this is unusually low, contamination with carbohydrate or protein should be suspected.
The usual method of analysis is the Zeisel procedure, whereby
the lignin is refluxed with hydriodic acid to yield the methyl
iodide which can be determined titrimetrically. A detailed
description of methods and apparatus is given in references
(2, 17 84). A colorimetric procedure has been described by
Mathers and Pro (61). The methoxyl groups are split off as
methanol after refluxing with concentrated sulfuric acid.
The methanol is oxidized to formaldehyde which is determined
colorimetrically after condensation with chromotropic acid.
Potentially, the methanol could also be determined by gas
chromatography, which would considerably facilitate the procedure.

Pectin and some other nonlignin compounds contain methoxyl groups, so the methoxyl content of the whole plant is
not a good indication of its lignin content.

The purity of the lignin preparation is also reflected
in its elemental composition. A variety of gas chromato-
graphs are at present available for determining C, H, N,
O, S and halogens. The subject has been reviewed by Rezl
and Janák (78). Oxygen can be estimated by difference. In
most purified lignins except Klason lignins, the proportion
of ash is usually insignificant, while the S content is only
important in the case of lignothioglycolic acids or if protein contamination is high. Sulfur can be very easily determined by the oxygen flash method described by Macdonald (57).

In neutral solvents, ultraviolet spectra of lignins
show a single peak at about 280 nm and, if ester groups are
present such as in grass MWL, a second peak at 315 nm is
observed. With the same lignin in alkali solution, the band
originally at 280 nm may be shifted to slightly longer wave-
lengths (280 to 290 nm) but that originally at 315 nm is
shifted to 355 nm (42). Ultraviolet difference spectra have
been used to measure the content of phenolic hydroxyl groups.
These ionize in alkaline solutions causing a change in the
extinction coefficient that is proportional to the number of

phenolic hydroxyl groups (3, 31). In the difference spectrum, maxima are found at 250 nm and 300 nm for the phenolic ions of simple substituted aromatic hydroxyl compounds, and at 250 and 350 nm for phenolic compounds in which the hydroxyl group is conjugated through the ring with a carbonyl group in the sidechain(31). Wexler (102) obtains the percentage of phenolic hydroxyl groups by multiplying the difference absorptivity (in liters/g.cm) at 250 nm by 0.192. This factor was obtained by dividing the percentage phenolic hydroxyl of four nonconjugated, phenolic, guaiacol compounds by their difference absorptivities at 250 nm. He also measured the absorption from a base line connecting the two minima on either side of the peak at about 230 nm and 280 nm. In Goldschmid's method, the difference absorptivity is measured at 300 nm and multiplied by a factor of 0.414 to give the percent phenolic hydroxyl.

The infrared spectra of various lignin preparations appear to be very similar, apart from differences in the relative intensities of the absorption bonds. Bands at about 1600 and 1500 cm^{-1} are especially characteristic of lignin. Kawamura and Higuchi (46) made an intensive study of the infrared spectra of MWL from various taxonomic classes of the plant kingdom and showed that various plant classes could be identified from their infrared spectra.

The proton magnetic spectra (PMR) of lignins indicate the distribution of the protons in the lignin molecule. The classical study has been made by Ludwig et al. (56). One problem is finding suitable solvents to dissolve some lignins. Many lignins are insoluble in CDCl$_3$ or other common PMR solvents and need prior acetylation. Dimethylsulfoxide is a good solvent but even the deuterated (99.9%) solvent shows a significant peak because of the solvent itself (33). A number of different solvents were compared by Lenz (54).

Recently (55) carbon-13 nuclear magnetic resonance spectra have been obtained for beech and spruce and the various peaks assigned to functional groups by comparison with model compounds. The technique offers considerable potential with the increasing availability of ^{13}C NMR spectrophotometers.

   Molecular weight distribution of lignin preparations
can now be easily determined using gel-chromatographic
procedures (47, 85). Values range from less than 1000 to
over 1 million, and any single preparation is usually poly-
disperse (35). The polydispersity probably arises from rup-
ture of chemical bonds during solvent extraction. Extraction of spruce lignin with solvents containing an acid
catalyst cleaves the five benzyl ethers in every eighteen
phenylpropane units (Figure 3), forming linear or slightly
branched lignin units (6).

   The above review has covered briefly some of the major
techniques used for characterizing lignins, but a variety
of other chemical procedures have been used. For further
details the reader is referred to the volumes by Brauns (9),
Brauns and Brauns (10), Freudenberg and Neish (27), and that
edited by Sarkanen and Ludwig (79).

              V.   EFFECT OF DIGESTION ON LIGNIN

   Such is the apparent indigestibility of lignin that it
is often used by animal scientists as a marker to predict
the apparent digestibility of a feed sample from a knowledge
of the concentration of the lignin in the feed and the feces
according to the following equation:

$$\text{Apparent digestibility } (\%) = \left[1 - \frac{\% \text{ lignin in food}}{\% \text{ lignin in feces}} \right] \times 100$$

This assumes that the digestibility of lignin is zero. However, the review by Streeter (92) shows that the recovery
of ingested lignin from ruminant feces varies from 50% to
over 100%. In the latter case, the method of analysis is at
fault, but there is a real possibility that some lignin is
made soluble upon digestion. This is supported by the fact
that a greater proportion of the total lignin (measured as
Klason lignin) is extractable with alkali from feces than
from the corresponding feed sample (32). It is unlikely
that significant enzymic digestion of lignin occurs, but
removal of neighboring carbohydrates may increase its solubility. It is possible that changes in pH along the digestive tract release portions of the lignin molecule or alter
functional groups. Ester and benzyl- and β-ether bonds
would be split the most readily.

Differences between the food and feces in the yields of the products upon alkaline nitrobenzene oxidation have been reported (7, 20, 75). Bondi and Meyer (7) showed that digestion resulted in the loss of nonphenolic hydroxyl groups and ethanolysis products, soluble in bisulfite. The last fact suggests a loss of arylglycerol-β-ether links since the bisulfite soluble fraction contains Hibbert's ketones. Ferulic and to a lesser extent p-coumaric acids are also lost upon digestion, but whether they are absorbed as such or merely structurally altered is not clear (34, 39). A loss of methoxyl groups upon digestion has been reported (19, 76), but this is not always so (7, 32). This discrepancy may be due to differences in the type of plant material used. Aerobic decomposition of lignin occurs through the action of phenol oxidases secreted by soil micro-organisms and fungi (37) but such a breakdown is unlikely in the anaerobic conditions of the gut. Harkin (37) has suggested the possibility of microbial etherases, which could split arylglycerol-β-aryl ethers and methyl aryl ethers, and it is possible that rumen fluid may contain such an enzyme. However, a loss in methoxyl groups would also occur through removal of portions of the lignin which have a high proportion of syringyl groups. Based on ultraviolet analyses of forage lignins before and after digestion, Allinson and Osbourn (1) suggested that simple nonconjugated phenolic units were degraded to some extent in the rumen.

Were significant absorption of lignin fragments occurring, one might expect an increase in the proportion of aromatic compounds excreted in the urine. This was studied in sheep by Martin (60), whose work indicates that other nonlignin phenolic compounds in ruminant food contributes to the urinary content of aromatic compounds.

Negative digestibilities of lignin can result from the formation of "artifact" lignin during digestion. The lignin in sainfoin showed negative digestibilities for sheep as high as -76% (1). During digestion a chemical fraction that analyzed as lignin and absorbed at a wavelength typical of nonconjugated phenols was produced in the intestinal digesta. Underestimating the lignin content in the undigested feed will also result in negative digestibility coefficients for lignin.

VI. LIGNIN CONTENT OF HUMAN FOODS

About 100 food items of vegetable origin were analyzed
for their content of Klason lignin at the University of
Guelph, Canada. This study showed that the intake of lignin
by humans is probably less than 2 to 3 g/day. The highest
concentrations of lignin are found in the breakfast cereals
(average 1% fresh weight) followed by fruit and vegetables
(0.2% fresh weight for each). A variety of fresh breads
contained only about 0.1% Klason lignin, and potatoes contained only about 0.05%.

VII. SUMMARY

Lignin is a substance found in the cell walls of plants
intimately associated with cellulose and hemicellulose. It
is probably the least digestible component of plants and also
depresses the digestibility of the cell-wall carbohydrates.
Its proportion increases as the plants age, thus contribut-
ing to their decline in digestibility.

Chemically, lignin is a three-dimensional aromatic
copolymer. In spruce wood it apparently arises by dehydrogenation of a mixture of 80% coniferyl alcohol, 14% p-coumaryl
alcohol, and 6% sinapyl alcohol. Lignins from grasses also
contain substantial amounts of p-coumaric and ferulic acids
esterified to the main lignin core. In grasses ferulic acid
may also constitute part of the core lignin.

Some and perhaps most of the lignin is chemically linked
to hemicellulose, and there may be some linkages with cellulose as well. The nature of these linkages has not been
established.

Lignin is quite insoluble in acids but substantial
amounts may be dissolved by alkali. It is partially soluble
in certain solvents such as dioxane. This solubility is
increased by ball-milling the sample and by the presence of
small amounts of water. Milled wood lignins obtained in
this manner are thought to be the nearest representative of
lignin as it exists in situ, but not all of the lignin is
extracted. Thioglycolic acid is thought to extract most of
the lignin, but allowance must be made for the incorporation
of this acid into the lignin. Alkali lignins have been recommended for studying grass lignins.

The usual method of estimating total lignin in herbaceous plants is to first subject the material to pretreatments, which remove firstly the cell contents (especially
protein) and then hemicellulose. The lignin-plus-cellulose
residue is then treated with 72% sulfuric acid to remove
cellulose, leaving a residue of Klason lignin plus ash.

Histochemically, the Wiesner and Maüle reactions are
common staining techniques for lignin. The latter distinguishes between hard and softwood lignins.

Purified lignins or lignin in situ can be degraded by
a variety of techniques to yield monomeric products, which
give some idea of the chemical makeup of the lignin. Alkaline nitrobenzene oxidation results in a loss of the propane
sidechain structure, but the ethanolysis and acidolysis procedures do not.

The methoxyl and elemental content of lignins are
important analytical features of lignin. A variety of
physical methods can also be used to characterize lignin
including ultraviolet, infrared, and nuclear magnetic resonance spectroscopy.

Although no intestinal enzymes capable of degrading
lignin of endogenous or exogenous origin have been demonstrated, intestinal dissolution of some lignin can occur
with some plants, and both hydroxyl and/or methoxyl groups
may be lost or altered upon digestion. Ferulic and p-coumaric
acids disappear upon digestion.

The lignin intake by humans is probably less than 2 to
3 g/day. The foods with the highest concentration of lignin
are the breakfast cereals. Potatoes and most breads are
very low in lignin, while fruits and vegetables have intermediate contents.

REFERENCES

1.   Allinson, D. W., and Osbourne, D. F., 1970, The cellu-
     lose-lignin complex in forages and its relationship to
     forage nutritive value, J. Agric. Sci., 74:23.

2. Association of Official Analytical Chemists, Official
    methods of analysis, edited by W. Horowitz, eleventh
    edition, 1970, p. 862.

3. Aulin-Erdtmann, G., 1952, Spectrographic contributions
    to lignin chemistry, II, Svensk Papperstindning,
    55:745.

4. Bjorkman, A., 1956, Studies on finely divided wood, I,
    Svensk Papperstidning, 59:477.

5. Bjorkman, A., 1957, Studies on finely divided wood,
    III, Svensk Papperstidning, 60:243.

6. Bolker, H. I., and Brenner, H. S., 1970, Polymeric
    structure of spruce lignin, Science, 170:173.

7. Bondi, A., and Meyer, H., 1948, Lignins in young plants,
    Biochem. J., 43:248.

8. Brand, J. M., 1967, Studies on grass lignins, II. The
    estimation of lignin oxidation products by gas-liquid
    chromatography, J. Chromatog., 26:373.

9. Brauns, F. E., The Chemistry of Lignin (New York:
    Academic Press, 1952).

10. Brauns, F. E., and Brauns, D. A., The Chemistry of
    Lignin, supplement volume (New York: Academic, 1960).

11. Brown, S. A., Biochemistry of Phenolic Compounds,
    J. B. Harborne, editor (London: Academic, 1964),
    chapter 9, p. 361.

12. Brown, S. A., 1966, Lignins, Ann. Review of Plant
    Physiol., 17:223.

13. Brown, S. A., 1969, Biochemistry of lignin formation,
    BioScience, 19:115.

14. Brownell, H. H., 1965, Isolation of milled wood lignin
    and lignin-carbohydrate complex, TAPPI, 48:513.

15. Brownell, H. H., 1968, Improved ball milling in the iso-
    lation of milled wood lignin, TAPPI, 51:298.

16. Chang, H. M., and Allan, G. G., "Oxidation," in:
Lignins, Occurrence, Formation, Structure and Reactions,
K. V. Sarkanen and C. H. Ludwig, editors, (New York:
Wiley Interscience, 1971) chapter 11, p. 433.

17. Clark. E. P., 1932, The Vieböck and Schwappach method
for the determination of methoxyl and ethoxyl groups,
J. A. O. A. C., 15:136.

18. Creighton, R. H. J., and Hibbert, H., 1944, Studies on
lignin and related compounds, LXXVI. Alkaline nitrobenzene oxidation of corn stalks. Isolation of p-hydroxybenzaldehyde, J. Amer. Chem. Soc., 66:37.

19. Csonka, F. A., Phillips, M. and Jones, D. B., 1929,
Studies on lignin metabolism, J. Biol. Chem., 85:65.

20. Cymbaluk, N. F., Gordon, A. J., and Neudoerffer, T. S.,
1973, The effect of the chemical composition of maize
plant lignin on the digestibility of maize stalk in
the rumen of cattle, Br. J. Nutr., 29:1.

21. Cymbaluk, N. F., and Neudoerffer, T. S., 1970, A quantitative gas-liquid chromatographic determination of
aromatic aldehydes from nitrobenzene oxidation of lignin, J. Chromatog., 54:167.

22. Donnelly, E. D., and Wear, J. I., 1972, Acid detergent
method for reduction of tannin interference in determining lignin of Sericea Lespediza, Agron. J., 64:838.

23. Edwards, C. S., 1973, Determination of lignin and cellulose in forages by extraction with triethylene glycol,
J. Sci. Fd. Agric., 24:381.

24. El-Basyouni, S. Z., and Towers, G. H. N., 1964, The
phenolic acids in wheat, I. Changes during growth and
development, Can. J. Biochem., 42:203.

25. Ellis, G. H., Matrone, G., and Maynard, L. A., 1946,
A 72-percent H_2SO_4 method for the determination of
lignin and its use in animal nutrition studies, J. Anim.
Sci., 5:285.

26. Fischer, H., 1961, Quantitative determination of lignin
     in hay, Acta Agric. Scand., Supplementum Number 10,
     43 p.

27. Freudenberg, K., 1964, Lignin: Its constitution and
     formation from p-hydroxycinnamyl alcohols, Science,
     148:595.

28. Freudenberg, K., in: Constitution and Biosynthesis of
     Lignin, by K. Freudenberg and A. C. Neish, (New York:
     Springer, 1968) p. 47.

29. Gee, M., Nelson, O. E., and Kuć, J., 1968, Abnormal
     lignins produced by the Brown-Midrib Mutants of maize,
     II, Archs. Biochem. Biophys., 123:403.

30. Gierer, J., 1954, Die reaktion von Chinonmonochlorimid
     mit lignin, I. Spezifitat der reaktion auf p-Oxybenzyl-
     alkoholgruppen und der Bestimmung in verschiedenen
     Ligninpräparaten, Acta Chemica Scand., 8:1319.

31. Goldschmid, O., 1954, Determination of phenolic hydroxyl
     content of lignin preparations by ultraviolet spectro-
     photometry, Anal. Chem., 26:1421.

32. Gordon, A. J., A comparison of some chemical and physi-
     cal properties of alkali ligning from grass and lucerne
     hays before and after digestion by sheep, J. Sci. Fd.
     Agric., in press.

33. Gordon, A. J., and Griffith, P. R., 1973, Chemical and
     in vivo evaluation of a Brown Midrib Mutant of Zea mays,
     II. Nuclear magnetic resonance spectra of digested and
     undigested alkali lignins and undigested dimethylforma-
     tide lignins, J. Sci. Fd. Agric., 24:579.

34. Gordon, A. J., and Neudoerffer, T. S., Chemical and in
     vivo evaluation of a Brown Midrib Mutant of Zea mays,
     I. Fibre, lignin and amino acid composition and di-
     gestibility for sheep, J. Sci. Fd. Agric., 24:565, 1973.

35. Goring, D. A. I., "Polymer properties of lignin and
     lignin derivatives," in: Lignins, Occurrence, Formation,
     Structure, and Reactions, K. V. Sarkanen and C. H.
     Ludwig, editors, (New York: Wiley Interscience, 1971)
     chapt. 17, p. 695.

36. Hall, F. K., 1974, Wood pulp, Scientific American, 230:51.

37. Harkin, J. M., 1967,"Lignin - a natural polymeric product of phenol oxidation," in: Oxidative Coupling of Phenols, edited by W. I. Taylor and A. R. Battersby, New York: Marcel Dekker, Inc., chapter 6, p. 243.

38. Hartley, R. D., 1971, Improved methods for the estimation by gas-liquid chromatography of lignin degradation products from plants, J. Chromatog., 54:335.

39. Hartley, R. D., 1972, p-Coumaric and ferulic acid components of cell walls of ryegrass and their relationships with lignin and digestibility, J. Sci. Fd. Agric., 23:1347.

40. Hartley, R. D., 1973, Carbohydrate esters of ferulic acid as components of cell walls of Lolium multiflorum, Phytochem., 12:661.

41. Higuchi, T., Ito, Y., and Kawamura, I., 1967, p-Hydroxyphenylpropane component of grass lignin and role of tryosine-ammonia lyase in its formation, Phytochem, 6:875.

42. Higuchi, T., Ito, Y., Shimada, M., and Kawamura, I., 1967, Chemical properties of milled wood lignin of grasses, Phytochem., 6:1551.

43. Higuchi, T., and Kawamura, I., 1966, Occurrence of p-hydroxyphenylglycerol-β-aryl ether structure in lignins, Holzforschung, 20:16.

44. Higuchi, T., Tanahashi, M., and Sato, A., 1972, Acidolysis of bamboo lignin, I. Gas-liquid chromatography and mass spectrometry of acidolysis monomers, Mokuzai Gakkaishi, 18:183.

45. Johnson, D. B., Moore, W. E., and Zank, L. C., 1961, The spectrophotometric determination of lignin in small wood samples, TAPPI, 44:793.

46. Kawamura, I. and Higuchi, T., 1964, Comparative studies
     of milled wood lignins from different taxonomical ori-
     gins by infrared spectroscopy, in: Chimie et Biochimie
     de la lignine, de la cellulose et des hemicelluloses,
     Symp., Grenoble, p. 439.

47. Kirk, T. K., Brown, W., and Cowling, E. B., 1969,
     Preparative fractionation of lignin by gel-permeation
     chromatography, Biopolymers, 7:135.

48. Košíková, B., and Polčin, J., 1973, Isolation of lignin
     from spruce by acidolysis in dioxane, Wood Science and
     Technology, 7:308.

49. Kuć, J., and Nelson, O. E., 1964, The abnormal lignins
     produced by the brown-midrib mutants of maize, I,
     Archs. Biochem. Biophys., 105:103.

50. Kuć, J., Nelson, O. E., and Flanagan, P., 1968, Degrada-
     tion of abnormal lignins in the Brown-Midrib Mutants
     and Double Mutants of maize, Phytochem., 7:1435.

51. Kutscha, N. P., and Gray, J. R., 1970, The potential of
     lignin research, Technical Bulletin 41, Maine Agricul-
     tural Experiment Station, University of Maine, 20 pages.

52. Lai, Y. Z., and Sarkanen, K. V., "Isolation and struc-
     tural studies," in: Lignins, Occurrence, Formation,
     Structure and Reactions (New York: Wiley Interscience,
     1971) chapter 5, p. 165.

53. Leary, G., 1971, The problem of lignin, J. N. Z. Inst.
     Chem., 35:7.

54. Lenz, B. L., 1968, Application of nuclear magnetic
     resonance spectroscopy to characterization of lignin,
     TAPPI, 51:511.

55. Lüdemann, H. D., and Nimz, H., 1973, Carbon-13 nuclear
     magnetic resonance spectra of lignins, Biochem. Biophys.
     Res. Comm., 52:1162.

56. Ludwig, C. G., Nist, B. J., and McCarthy, J. L., 1963,
     Lignin, XII and XIII, J. Am. Chem. Soc., 86:1186 and
     1196.

57. Macdonald, A. M. G., "The oxygen-flash method," in: Advances in Analytical Chemistry and Instrumentation, C. N. Reilley, editor (New York: John Wiley and Sons, Inc.,1965) vol. 4, p. 75.

58. McKenzie, A. W., McPherson, J. A., and Stewart, C. M., 1955, The estimation of acid-soluble lignin, Holzforshung, 9:109.

59. Manning, K. R., and DeLong, W. A., 1941, The lignin content of some common vegetables with observations on methods for the determination of lignin, Sci. Agric., 22:69.

60. Martin, A. K., 1970, The urinary aromatic acids excreted by sheep given S24 perennial ryegrass cut at six stages of maturity, Br. J. Nutr., 24:943.

61. Mathers, A. P., and Pro, M. J., 1955, Spectrophotometric determination of methoxyl, Anal. Chem., 27:1662.

62. Merewether, J. W. T., 1957, A lignin-carbohydrate complex in wood, Holzforschung, 11:65.

63. Meyer, H., and Bondi, A., 1952, Lignin in young plants, Biochem. J., 52:95.

64. Miksche, G. E., 1973, Studies on the structure of gynmosperm and angiosperm lignins, Abstracts of Gothenburg Dissertations in Science, 31: 24 pages.

65. Moon, F. E., and Abou-Raya, A. K., 1954, The lignin fraction of animal feeding-stuffs, IV. The preparation of "Reference" lignin by extraction with ethyl acetoacetate, J. Sci. Fd. Agric., 5:319.

66. Morrison, I. M., 1972, Improvements in the acetyl bromide technique to determine lignin and digestibility and its application to legumes, J. Sci. Fd. Agric., 23:1463.

67. Morrison, I. M., 1974, Structural investigation on the lignin-carbohydrate complexes of Lolium perenne, Biochem. J., 139:197.

68. Neish, A. C., "Monomeric intermediates in the biosynthesis of lignin," in: Constitution and Biosynthesis of Lignin, by K. Freudenberg and A. C. Neish, (New York: Springer, 1968) p. 1.

69. Neth. J. Agric. Sci., 1966, 14:215.

70. Nimz, H., 1973, Chemistry of potential chromophoric groups in beech lignin, TAPPI, 56:124.

71. Pepper, J. M., and Wood, P. D. S., 1962, The isolation of a representative lignin fraction from wood and straw meals, Can. J. Chem., 40:1026.

72. Pepper, J. M., Manolopoulo, M., and Burton, R., 1962, Gas-liquid chromatographic analysis of lignin oxidation products, Can. J. Chem., 40:1976.

73. Pew, J. C., and Connors, W. J., 1969, New structures from enzymic dehydrogenation of lignin model p-hydroxy-propiophenones, J. Org. Chem., 34:585.

74. Phillips, M., Goss, M. J., Davis, B. L., and Stevens, H., 1939, Composition of the various parts of the oat plant at successive stages of growth, with special reference to the formation of lignin, Sci. Agric., 59:319.

75. Pigden, W. J., and Stone, J. E., 1952, The effect of ruminant digestion on forage lignin, Sci. Agric., 32:502.

76. Porter, P., and Singleton, A. G., 1971, The degradation of lignin and quantitative aspects of ruminant digestion, Br. J. Nutr., 25:3.

77. Quicke, G. V., and Bentley, O. G., 1959, Lignin and methoxyl as related to the decreased digestibility of mature forages, J. Anim. Sci., 18:365.

78. Rezl, V., and Janák, J., 1973, Elemental analysis by gas chromatography, J. Chromatog., 81:233.

79. Roadhouse, F. E. and MacDougall, D., 1956, A study of the nature of plant lignin by means of alkaline nitrobenzene oxidation, Biochem. J., 63:33,

80. Sarkanen, K. V., and Ludwig, C. H., editors, Lignins, Occurrence, Formation, Structure and Reactions, (New York: Wiley Interscience. 1971).

81. Sarkanen, K. V., "Precursors and their polymerization," in: Lignins, Occurrence, Formation, Structure and Reactions, K. V. Sarkanen and C. H. Ludwig, editors, (New York: Wiley Interscience, 1971), chapter 4, p. 95.

82. Sato, A., Nishio, K., and Kitamura, T., 1972, On the ratio of syringaldehyde to vanillin (S/V value) of the lignin in peanuts (Arachis hypogaea L.), Ag. Chem. (Japan), 46:603.

83. Shimada, M., 1972, Biochemical studies of bamboo lignin and methoxylation in hardwood and softwood lignins, Wood Research, 53:19.

84. Siggia, S., 1966, Quantative Organic Analysis via Functional Groups, third edition, New York: John Wiley and Sons, Inc., chapter 4, p. 209.

85. Soundararajan, T. N., and Wayman, M., 1970, The determination of the molecular weight and molecular weight distribution of dehydrogenase polymers of coniferyl alcohol and lignins, J. Polymer Sci., 30:521.

86. Stafford, H. A., 1960, Differences between lignin-like polymers formed by peroxidation of eugenol and ferulic acid in leaf sections of Phleum, Plant Physiol., 35:108.

87. Stafford, H. A., 1960, Comparison of lignin-like polymers produced peroxidatively by cinnamic acid derivatives in leaf sections of Phleum, Plant Physiol., 35:612.

88. Stafford, H. A., 1962, Histochemical and biochemical differences between lignin-like materials in Phleum pratense L., Plant Physiol., 37:643.

89. Stafford, H. A., 1964, Comparison of lignin-like
     products found naturally or induced in tissues of
     Phleum Elodea and Coleus and in a paper peroxidase
     system, Plant Physiol., 39:350.

90. Stafford, H. A., 1974, The metabolism of aromatic com-
     pounds, Ann. Review of Plant Physiol., 25:460.

91. Stone, J. E., Blundell, M. J., and Tanner, K. G., 1951,
     The formation of lignin in wheat plants, Can. J. Chem.,
     29:734.

92. Streeter, C. H., 1969, A review of techniques used to
     estimate the in vivo digestibility of grazed forage,
     J. Anim. Sci., 29:757.

93. Talmadge, K. W., Keegstra, K., Bauer, W. D., and
     Albersheim, P., 1973, The structure of plant cell
     walls, I, Plant Physiol., 51:158.

94. Thomas, B., and Armstrong, D. G., 1949, A study of some
     methods at present used for the determination of lignin,
     J. Agric. Sci., 39:335.

95. Van Soest, P. J., 1973, Use of detergents in the analy-
     sis of fibrous feeds, II. A rapid method for the deter-
     mination of fiber and lignin, J. A. O. A. C., 46:829.

96. Van Soest, P. J., 1964, Symposium on nutrition and for-
     age and pastures: New chemical procedures for evaluat-
     ing forages, J. Anim. Sci, 23:838.

97. Van Soest, P. J., 1967, Development of a comprehensive
     system of feed analyses and its application to forages,
     J. Anim. Sci., 26:119.

98. Van Soest, P. J., and McQueen, R. W., 1973, The chemis-
     try and estimation of fibre, Proc. Nutr. Soc., 32:123.

99. Van Soest, P. J., and Wine, R. H., 1967, Use of deter-
     gents in the analysis of fibrous feeds, IV. Determina-
     tion of plant cell-wall constituents, J. A. O. A. C.,
     50:50.

100. Van Soest, P. J. and Wine, R. H., 1968, Determination of lignin and cellulose in acid-detergent fiber with permanganate, J. A. O. A. C., 51:780.

101. Wardrop, A. B., "Occurrence and formation in plants," in: Lignins, Occurrence, Formation, Structure and Reactions, K. V. Sarkanen and C. H. Ludwig, editors, (New York: Wiley Interscience, 1971) chapter 2, p. 79.

102. Wexler, A. S., 1964, Characterization of lignosulfonates by ultraviolet spectrometry, Anal. Chem., 36:213.

103. Whitehead, D. L., and Quicke, G. V., 1960, The nitrogen content of grass lignin, J. Sci. Fd. Agric., 11:151.

CHAPTER 4

PECTIN

Lorne A. Campbell and Grant H. Palmer

Sunkist Growers

Ontario, California

I.   CHEMISTRY AND NOMENCLATURE

Pectic substances originate primarily in the cell walls and fibrous portions of fruit, vegetable, and other land plant tissues. They are complex colloidal carbohydrate derivatives containing as their major structural feature acid polysaccharides composed primarily of galaturonic acid units. Neutral sugars such as arabinose, galactose, rhamnose, and xylose have been identified as associated with the pectin molecule (1). Aspinall's work indicates that the rhamnose may be a part of the main chain structure of the pectin molecule. The association of arabinose and galactose may be either a sidechain attachment or an incidental part of the main chain. By this it is meant that the entire sugar molecule is not involved in the chain structure.

Part of the plant pectins are readily extracted with water. This readily soluble pectin in fruits increases as the fruit matures. The water-insoluble portion is known as protopectin, which consists of pectin bound with other tissue constituents, such as cellulose, to give rigidity to the tissue structure. Pectin will be released from protopectin by prolonged hydrolysis with hot water, by treatment with mild acid or alkali, by enzymes, and by holding at about 90°C in 0.5% ammonium oxalate.

The chemical extraction of pectin by these reagents has been illustrated by Joseph (8). (See Figure 1.)

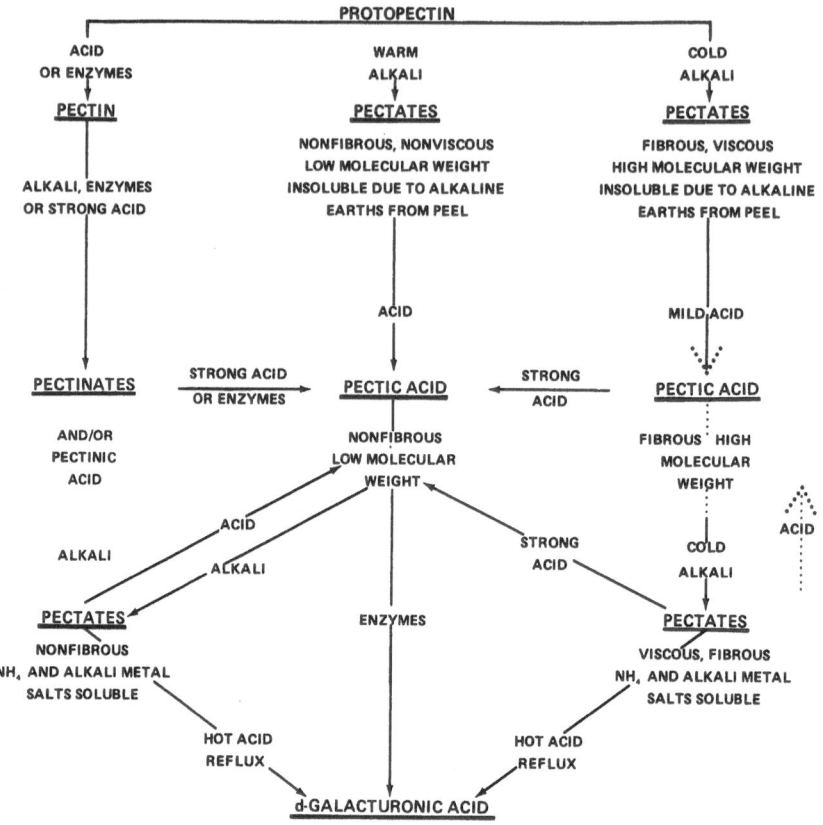

Figure 1.   Interrelationship of the pectic substances.   Reproduced with permission from Joseph (8).

When the carboxyl groups of the polygalacturonic acid chain are more than negligibly esterified by methyl groups, the term pectinic acid is applied.   The salts formed from partially esterified pectins are referred to as pectinates. Salts of the completely de-esterified pectin molecule are pectates.

A guide to pectin nomenclature was developed by Joseph (8).   Figure 2 comprises a nomenclature chart for pectic substances and the degrees (percentages) of esterification.

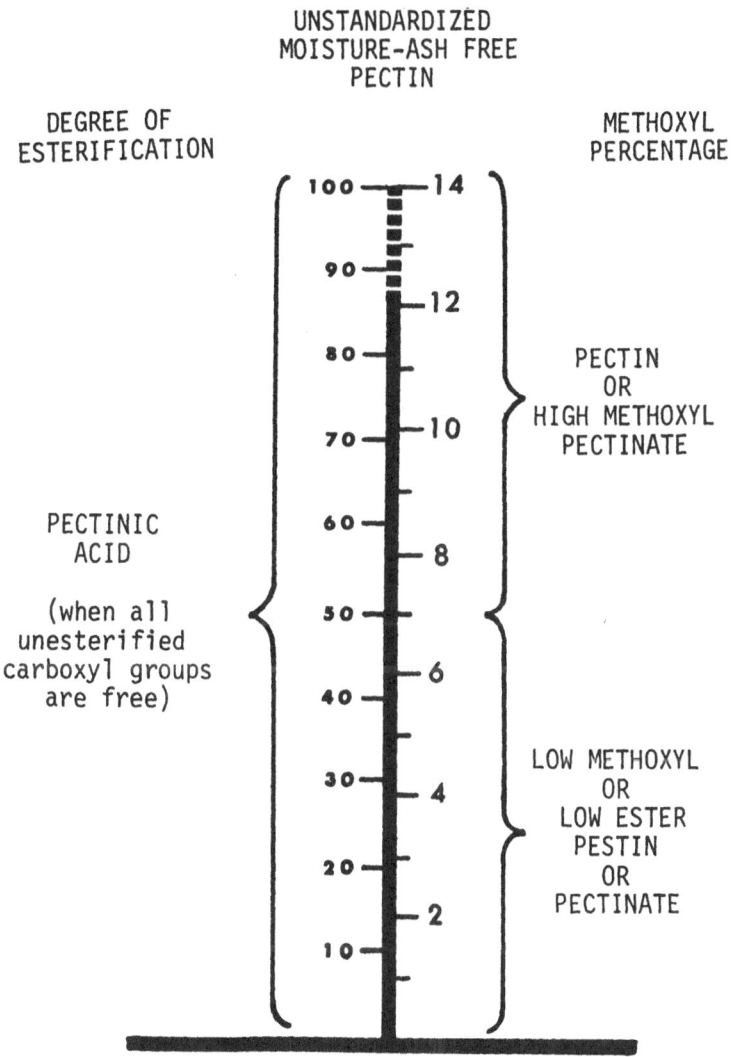

UNSTANDARDIZED
MOISTURE-ASH FREE
PECTIN

DEGREE OF   METHOXYL
ESTERIFICATION   PERCENTAGE

PECTIN
OR
HIGH METHOXYL
PECTINATE

PECTINIC
ACID

(when all
unesterified
carboxyl groups
are free)

LOW METHOXYL
OR
LOW ESTER
PESTIN
OR
PECTINATE

Figure 2.   Nomenclature chart for the pectic substances.

II. PECTIC ENZYMES

Pectic enzymes occur in a number of plants and micro-organisms and may be classified into pectin methylesterases and polygalacturonases. The pectin methylesterases hydrolyze the methylester linkages, whereas the polygalacturonases cleave the glycosidic bonds between the galacturonic acid molecules. Pectin transeliminases bring about the cleavage of the alpha (1→4) linkages, forming unsaturated derivatives of polygalacturonic acid. Recent work has shown that some of the pectic enzymes considered to be polygalacturonases may be reclassified as transliminases, since both these enzymes reduce the viscosity of pectin and produce a molecule of sugar for each alpha (1→4) linkage cleaved. Pectic enzymes can be subdivided further depending upon whether they act on the methylated or free polygalacturonic acid substances or whether they act on internal linkages. The pectic enzymes of commerce come from Aspergillus niger and are generally employed as a mixture of enzymes. Pectic enzymes may be added to a product to provide clarity or may be destroyed to preserve viscosity (17).

III. PECTIN CONTENT OF PLANT MATERIALS

Although pectins are found in the cell walls of all higher land plants, there is great variation in the pectic content of different plant varieties as well as in various plant materials. (See Table 1.) Of the various plant materials, one third of the dry weight of the albedo or white portion of citrus peel and 17% of dried apple pomace is pectin. From these two sources the major portion of commercial pectin is produced today.

IV. GEL FORMATION

A well-known characteristic of pectin is its ability to form jelly in the presence of acid and sugar. As discussed previously, the carboxyl groups of the polygalacturonic acids may be partially esterified by methyl groups as in pectinic acid. It is the degree of esterification that provides the name for the high-ester or high-methoxyl (HM) and distinguishes them from the low-ester or low-methoxyl (LM) pectins of commerce.

TABLE 1.   PECTIN CONTENT OF FRUITS AND VEGETABLES
(percent of fresh weight as calcium pectate)

Plant variety	%
Apples	0.71 - 0.84
Apricots	0.71 - 1.32
Asparagus	Trace
Bananas	0.59 - 1.28
Beans	0.27 - 1.11
Blackberries	0.68 - 1.19
Carrots	1.17 - 2.92
Cherries	0.24 - 0.54
Cucumbers	0.10 - 0.50
Dewberries	0.51 - 1.00
Grapes	0.09 - 0.28
Grapefruit	3.30 - 4.50
Lemons	2.80 - 2.99
Loganberries	0.59
Oranges	2.34 - 2.38
Raisins	0.82 - 1.04
Raspberries	0.97
Squash	1.00 - 2.00
Sweet potatoes	0.78

Although both types of commercial pectins will form
the pectin-sugar-acid jellies, gelation occurs under different conditions. The high-methoxyl or typical commercial
pectin, in order to form gels, must meet two requirements.
First, the sugar content or soluble solids level must be
over 50% of the weight of material in the preparation, and
second, the acid level must be adjusted to pH 2.9 to 3.4
depending on whether the pectin is rapid or slow setting.

Low-ester or low-methoxyl pectins, on the other hand,
form gels when an alkaline earth cation, usually calcium,
is included in the gel media. Sugar is not required in manu-
facturing gelled products using the low-ester pectin, and
this pectin forms suitable gels over a pH range of 2.5 to
6.5. Despite the fact that pectin was discovered before
the turn of the eighteenth century and has been used both
in the home and commercially for jelly manufacture for count-

less years, the exact mechanism of gel formation is still
not fully understood.

V. PECTIN METABOLISM

Experimental work on rats, dogs and man reveals that
pectin does not appear to be absorbed by these species.
A feeding trial carried out on weanling rats (18) using
0%, 5%, and 10% citrus pectin-S (55% esterified) and 10%
citrus pectin-M (65% esterified) showed that 100% of the
undigested compound could be recovered in the feces of
these animals. Galacturonic acid, a metabolite of pectin,
was not absorbed in any appreciable quantities from the
human or canine ileum or the canine colon (19). Pectin
administered to dogs passed through the stomach and part of
the small intestine and was recovered without loss (9).

Kertesz reported that saliva and gastric juice do not
act enzymatically on pectin (9). Nor did in-vitro studies
with trypsin and pepsin reveal any hydrolytic effect of
these intestinal enzymes on pectin. However, pectin incubated with fecal material is rapidly digested. Bacteria
capable of metabolizing pectin in vitro were isolated from
dog feces when the animal was fed pectin as its sole dietary
item for one week (20). The more active bacteria belonged
to aerobacillus, lactobacillus, micrococcus, and entero-
coccus. Berkefeld filtrates of these organisms were shown
to contain heat-labile, pectinase-like enzymes, liquefying
enzymes and/or pectase-like, coagulating enzyme. Some
galacturonic acid and formic and acetic acids were the chief
products.

The definitive studies in man (19), using the ileos-
tomy technique, demonstrated that pectin is decomposed
chiefly in the colon and that bacterial rather than animal
enzymes are involved. Detailed studies carried out in the
rat (6) showed that apple pectin is attacked by the intestinal flora and metabolized into galacturonic acid, other organic acids that are capable of resorption, and finally
carbon dioxide and water.

Much controversy surrounds the values proposed for the
digestible energy of pectin. In a study with rats fed citrus pectin-S and pectin-M at dietary levels of 5 and 10%,

Viola (18) calculated the apparent digestible energy of
pectin. In these experiments the contribution of pectin-M
and pectin-S were both negative and were reported as -1.60
and -1.65 kcal/g, respectively.

Viola's work substantiated earlier work carried out
by the Western Regional Research Laboratories in California
(3). These workers fed 10% of citrus pectin to rats and
concluded that this material was apparently not utilized by
the rat. They based their conclusions on the fact that
practically all the pectin fed could be accounted for in
the feces.

In opposition to these two studies is the one carried
out by Gaedeken (6) on the rat using apple pectin at dietary
levels of 12.0 and 23.7%. Calculations from these studies
showed a digestible energy which was calculated to 3.55 and
3.48 kcal for the 12.0-and 23.7-% dietary levels, respectively. Calculations from studies carried out in Sunkist
Laboratories (15) using low-meth-oxy pectin and Pectin N.F.
administered to human volunteers at a dosage level of 5 g
3x/day with meals showed the digestible energy of these
compounds to be 2.86 kcal/g and 3.03 kcal/g, respectively.

Besides the numerous uses of pectin in food products,
much work has been carried out to study the hypocholesterolemic activity of this material both in man and laboratory
animals. In a 4-week study, Fisher et al.(5) noted a hypocholesterolemic activity in pigs. Four groups of each sex
of Yorkshire pigs 8 weeks of age or four Hampshire pigs 16
weeks old were fed 5% pectin or 5% cellulose in a diet with
and without cholesterol. Swine on the pectin-plus-choles-
terol diet showed a lowering of their serum cholesterol
levels when compared to those animals on a cholesterol-free
diet. These trials suggest that an exogenous dietary source
of cholesterol is necessary for the lowering of serum cholesterol in this experimental animal.

A 28-day study was carried out by Leveille and Sauberlich (12) in male rats fed 1% cholesterol with or without
pectin. Those animals fed pectin showed a lowering of
plasma and liver cholesterol. In-vitro studies revealed that
pectin decreased by approximately 50% the transport of tauro-
cholic acid. Similar results were noted in vivo when pectin
and cholestyramine, an inhibitor of bile acid transport, were

fed to rats. Radioactive studies utilizing cholesterol-4-C^{14} in male Wistar rats showed that oral pectin reduced the absorption of the labeled cholesterol by 7% from control values (7).

Middle-aged men fed 15 g of citrus Pectin N.F. per day for several weeks had a decrease in their cholesterol levels of 5% below their control value (a 15-g cellulose diet) (11). Diets were similar in fats, cholesterol, and calories but differed in the carbohydrate source. A considerable amount of carbohydrate in one diet was provided by legumes. The other diet had this carbohydrate source matched by sugar. In both diets, citrus Pectin N.F. reduced the cholesterol level in the subjects under trial.

Palmer and Dixon (16) administered citrus Pectin N.F. orally to human volunteers. The pectin was administered in a randomized, double-blind program in capsules at 2-g increments including the same number of placebo capsules containing Alphacel®. The six 4-week test periods were followed by a 10-week period without treatment. Serum cholesterol levels were significantly reduced in 12 out of 16 of the test subjects when the daily intake was 6 or more g of pectin.

Other pharmacological studies have been carried out in laboratory animals to determine if pectin possesses other activities besides its effect on serum cholesterol. Citrus Pectin N.F. fed orally to rabbits reduced gallstone formation when compared with the controls (4). Other investigations have been carried out to study the antiulcer effect of plantaglucide, the powdered pectin from the leaves of the large plantain (14). Stomach ulcers were induced in rats by injecting phenylbutazone intramuscularly. The authors concluded that plantaglucide had a distinct antiulcer effect on this experimental animal.

Of considerable interest is the antidiarrheal effect of pectin in man. Much of the work in this area has been carried out by Bender (2), who hypothesizes that pectin moves rapidly to the large intestine, coating the mucosa with unchanged polysaccharide. There, it is used as a carbon source by the normal flora. In addition to D-galacturonic acid, lower organic acids, especially acetic and formic acids, are formed producing the normal complement of acids that sta-

bilize the pH of the colon. These acids are also bacterio-
static against most pathogens at normal bowel pH. Since
disorders associated with abnormal and undesirable flora
are usually accompanied by a higher-than-normal pH, the
inflow of pectin and the subsequent return to normal pH by
its digestion adversely affect the growth of the pathogens
and encourages the normal flora to return to full activity.

There are two apparent causes for this return to nor-
malcy: the lowering of pH and the production of certain acid
radicals at levels that cannot be tolerated by most of the
pathogens. However, some effects remain that are not explained by this mechanism, such as the extremely prompt but
usually only temporary relief that results from a single
dose, with the need of two or more doses for complete relief;
the almost immediate reversal of the fatigued feeling to one
of well-being, and the inhibiting effect of pectin on certain
viruses. The mechanism of the action of pectin as an antidiarrheal in man still requires much investigation.

VI. CONCLUSION

In 1951 Kertesz compiled most of the information that
was available on pectin to that date (10). The work reported
in this chapter shows that pectic substances have been and
remain a fascinating group of natural compounds. Of particular interest are the role that these materials play in the
daily dietary and the contribution they make to the nutritional component of fiber. Much work remains to determine
the role of pectin in the plant cell walls. An excellent
recent review by Nelson et al. (13) on commercially important
pectin substances shows that much research needs to be done
into the chemical structure of pectin. Certainly a great
deal of work is necessary to determine the absorption, metabolism, and excretion of pectin substances and their metabolites in man, and further metabolic studies to determine the
digestible energy of these natural colloids in the human
subject.

Pharmacological activity such as the chelation of certain heavy metals by pectin, hypocholesterolemia and the antidiarrheal effect of pectin are fruitful fields for further
studies in order to determine the role of pectin in the phar-
maceutical armamentarium.

REFERENCES

1. Aspinall, G. O., Craig, J. W. T., and Whyte, J. L.,
    1968, Lemon pectin, I. Fractionization and partial
    hydrolysis of water-soluble pectin, Carbohydrate Res.,
    7:442.

2. Bender, W. A., Whistler, R. L., and Bemiller, J. N.,
    Industrial Gum, (New York: Academic Press, 1959) p. 377.

3. Booth, A. N., Henrickson, A. P., and Deeds, F., 1963,
    Physiological effects of 3 microbial polysaccharides
    on rats, Tox. App. Pharm., 5:478.

4. Borgman, R. F., and Haselden, F. H., 1969, Cholelithia-
    sis in rabbits: effect of several treatments on forma-
    tion and dissolution of gallstones, Am. J. Vet. Res.,
    30:1979.

5. Fisher, H., Van der Noot, W., McGlath, W. S., and
    Grimiger, P., 1966, Dietary pectin and plasma cho-
    lesterol in swine, Atheroscler. Res., 6:190.

6. Gaedeken, D., 1969, Energetic evaluation of pectins in
    monogastrics, Landwirt. Forsch. Sonderh., 23:9.

7. Hyun, S. A., Vahouny, G. V., and Treadwell, C. R., 1963,
    Effect of hypocholesterolemic agents on intestinal cho-
    lesterol absorption, Proc. Soc. Exptl. Biol. Med., 112:
    496.

8. Joseph, G. H., "Pectic substances in the food industries,"
    in: Advances in Chemistry, No. 12 (Washington, D.C.:
    Am. Chem. Soc., 1955) p. 49.

9. Kertesz, Z. I., 1940, Pectic enzymes v. fate of pectins
    in the animal body, J. Nutrition, 20:289.

10. Kertesz, Z. I., The Pectic Substances (New York: Inter-
    science, 1951).

11. Keys, A., Grande, F., and Anderson, J. T., 1961, Fiber
    and pectin in the diet and serum cholesterol concentra-
    tion in man, Proc. Soc. Exptl. Biol. Med., 106:555.

12. Leveille, G. A., and Sauberlich, H. E., 1966, Mechanism of the cholesterol-depressing effect of pectin in the cholesterol-fed rat, J. Nutr., 88:209.

13. Nelson, D. B., Smit, Christian, J. B., and Wiles, R. R., "Commercially important pectic substances," in: Food Colloids, H. D. Graham, editor (Westport, Connecticut: Avi Publishing) in press.

14. Obolentseva, G. V., and Yai, K., 1966, Pharmacological analysis of plantaglucide, Moscow: Farmakol., 29:469.

15. Palmer, G. H., and Bryant, E. F., 1952, Preliminary studies of ingested pectins, report to Sunkist Growers, Inc., Research Department.

16. Palmer, G. H., and Dixon, O. G., 1966, Effect of pectin dose on serum cholesterol levels, Am. J. Clin. Nutr., 18:437.

17. Underkofler, L. A., "Enzymes," in: Handbook of Food Additives (Ohio: The Chemical Rubber Co., 1968) p. 51.

18. Viola, S., Zimmerman, G., and Mokady, S., 1970, Effect of pectin and algin upon protein utilization, digestibility of nutrients and energy in young rats, Nutr. Rep. Int., 1:367.

19. Werch, S. C., and Ivy, A. C., 1941, The fate of ingested pectin, Am. J. Digestive Diseases, 8:101.

20. Werch, S. C., Jung, R. W., Day, A. A., Friedman, T. E., and Ivy, A. C., 1942, The decomposition of pectin and galacturonic acid by intestinal bacteria, J. Infect. Dis., 70:231.

CHAPTER 5

PLANT FIBERS AND HUMAN HEALTH

Mervin G. H. Hardinge

Loma Linda University

Loma Linda, California

I. INTRODUCTION

Throughout the history of the nutritional science, attention has centered mainly on the nutrient requirements. Fats, proteins, carbohydrates, minerals, vitamins and the water intake have all come under close study in an effort to determine the body's need for each, the effect on health of a deficiency or an excess, and the quantitative interrelationships of nutrients.

During all this intense study of foods over the past century, the indigestible constituents of the diet have generally been considered of little consequence to health, if not actually undesirable. Thus by milling off the bran and germ of cereal grains, by extracting the sweet juices from sugar cane and sugar beets and concentrating them to pure crystals, and by extracting or pressing the oil from fat-rich seeds and olives, we have established a dietary pattern in the United States in which over 50% of the calories come from refined foods that contain little or no indigestible residue. The diets of other Western countries are similar.

II. DIETARY FIBER IN VEGETARIAN AND NONVEGETARIAN DIETS

In 1958, Hardinge et al. (6) studied the fiber content of the diets of 86 lacto-ovo-vegetarian, 26 "pure" vegetarian and 88 nonvegetarian adults, adolescents, and pregnant women. The nutritional, physical, and laboratory find-

ings were described previously (7). Lacto-ovo-vegetarians
include dairy products and eggs in their diets, but no flesh
of animals (meat, poultry, or fish). Pure vegetarians eat
no foods of animal origin. Their entire diet consists of
plant foods.

All the vegetarians of this study had maintained their
respective dietaries for long periods of time. With few
exceptions, the lacto-ovo-vegetarians had been lifetime
adherents and some had family histories of two to three
generations of vegetarianism. The pure-vegetarian males
averaged 16 years on their diets and the females 9 years;
the minimum was 5 years. All the subjects of the various
groups were in apparent good health.

Table 1 summarizes the crude fiber intake of our subjects as calculated by the use, mainly, of the Department
of Agriculture food composition tables (19). Crude fiber
values are considerably lower than the total indigestible
residue of food, for which no extensive tables are available.

As the table shows, the pure vegetarians consumed by
far the largest amount of plant fiber (males 23.9 g and
females 20.7 g), and the nonvegetarians the least (adult
males 10.7 g and adult females 8.4 g). The lacto-ovo-
vegetarians were intermediate (adult males 16.3 g and adult
females 12.8 g). The reason for this difference lies in the
nature of the dietary patterns followed. Not only did the
pure vegetarians live entirely on the product of the earth,
but their choice of plant foods included practically none of
the refined types so commonly used in conventional diets.
Their protein and calories were derived mainly from foods
rich in fiber, whole-grain cereals, legumes, nuts, and such
nutlike seeds as sunflower and sesame. Characteristic also
of this group was the consumption of unusually large amounts
of fruits, fresh, dried, and canned, and of vegetables, both
cooked and in the form of very large raw salads. Virtually
every food eaten contributed its share of fiber to the diet.

The nonvegetarian diets, on the other hand, although
highest in calories, were lowest in fiber content. Animal
protein--meat, milk, cheese, and eggs--all of which contain
little or no indigestible material, made up approximately
two thirds of their protein intake and about 30% of their
total calories. The lacto-ovo-vegetarians, whose dietary

Table 1. Comparison of Crude Fiber Intakes of Vegetarian and Nonvegetarian Groups

Groups	No.	kcal	g/day Mean	g/day S.D.[1]	Fiber mg/100kcal (mean)	mg/kg/body wt (mean)
Adults						
Males						
L-o-vegetarian[2]	15	3020	16.3	9.3	537	220
Pure vegetarian	14	3620	23.9	7.0	787	362
Nonvegetarian	15	3720	10.7	3.3	288	139
Females						
L-o-vegetarian	15	2450	12.6	9.3	515	201
Pure vegetarian	11	2400	20.7	7.3	857	390
Nonvegetarian	15	2690	8.4	1.9	313	131
Adolescent						
Males						
L-o-vegetarian	15	4450	17.8	8.2	399	278
Nonvegetarian	15	5350	12.2	3.2	228	192
Females						
L-o-vegetarian	15	3030	12.9	7.3	417	242
Nonvegetarian	15	4100	10.6	2.2	257	208
Pregnant Women						
L-o-vegetarian	26	2650	12.4	11.1	467	210
Nonvegetarian	28	3010	8.4	5.4	282	144

[1]Standard Deviation.   [2]Lacto-ovo-vegetarian.

pattern closely resembled the conventional American diet
except, mainly, for the absence of flesh foods, obtained
about half of their total protein and 20% of their total
calories from milk, cheese, and eggs. Their use of refined
cereal products and of commercially prepared foods, though
less than that of the nonvegetarians, was much more liberal
than that of the pure vegetarians. They also used larger
quantities of legumes, nuts, and whole-grain breads and
cereals, as well as more fruits and vegetables, than the
nonvegetarians. But since their diets included some fiber-
free and some low-fiber foods, their total intake of crude
fiber was significantly less than that of the pure vegetarians, although it considerably exceeded that of the nonvegetarians.

That the diets of vegetarians contain larger amounts
of indigestible carbohydrates than those of nonvegetarians
has also been observed by others. Kirkeby (12) did a study
of 116 Norwegian lacto-vegetarians among whom were a few
pure vegetarians. In comparison with the control group, the
vegetarian diet was judged to be "lower in sugar and higher
in complex carbohydrates, starches, pectins, and celluloses,
than the ordinary diet." One of the sources of fiber was
dark bread that retained a good proportion of the bran of the
whole grain.

West and Hayes (20) found a significantly higher fiber
intake among vegetarians of the Seventh-Day Adventist Church
than among members of the same church who did not adhere to
a vegetarian diet.

Both vegetarians who reject flesh foods by choice and
near-vegetarians who cannot afford to buy it or cannot obtain it are reported to consume large amounts of nonabsorbable carbohydrates. Burkitt et al. (2) found that the stools
of British vegetarians weighed twice as much, and those of
rural Ugandan villagers four times as much, as the stools of
English students and of young men of the Royal Navy.

III.   DIETARY FIBER AND EPIDEMIOLOGICAL ASPECT OF DISEASE

    A. Fiber Intake and Digestive System Function

Neither of our vegetarian groups reported any digestive
complaints due to the coarseness of their diets. Even the

large fiber intake of the pure vegetarians caused no alimentary disturbance. This is in keeping with the findings
of McCance et al. (14) in the feeding of brown bread made
from flour of 100% extraction. It also agrees with the
Danish experience during World War I. Under the direction
of Hindhede (10), who was given the task of rationing the
country's dwindling food supply during the blockade, Denmark
milled its rye to 100% and added to it some wheat bran and
whole-grain flour; the people suffered no digestive problems
and registered no complaints.

B.   Fiber Intake Effect on Character
and Transit Time of Stools

Unfortunately, the circumstances attending our investigation made it impractical to study the stools. However,
the level of fiber in the diets of even the nonvegetarians,
who consumed the least, was in excess of Cowgill's (4) estimated fiber requirement of 90 to 100 mg/kg body weight,
which amounts to approximately 6 g/day for an adult. There
was, therefore, no problem with constipation in any of our
groups. This finding is probably due to the fact that most
of our subjects resided in California, where fresh fruits
and vegetables are readily available throughout the year (2).

Burkitt and his coworker report that diets of high-fiber
intake produce stools that are large, soft, and nonodorous in
contrast to the consistency, size, and foul odor of the small,
firm stools of subjects in communities eating low-residue
diets. They found an inverse relationship between stool
weights and transit time and between fiber intake and transit
time. In the radiological study of the passage of brown and
white breads through the digestive tract, McCance and his
associates (14) observed that the brown bread residue left
the colon 24 hours sooner than that from the white bread.
Payler (16) fed 15- to 19-year-old boys whole meal bread
plus about 15 g of bran daily for three weeks, and mean stool
weight increased by 21% and transit time decreased by 29%.

C.   Fiber Intake and Body Weight

A comparison of the heights and weights of all our
groups of lifetime lacto-ovo-vegetarians and nonvegetarians
showed no significant differences. The pure vegetarians, how-

ever, both men and women, averaged 20 lbs less in weight
than their respective counterparts in the other two groups.
This was of interest in view of the fact that the caloric
intake of the pure vegetarians was approximately the same
as that of the other two groups, being slightly above that
of the lacto-ovo-vegetarians and not much less than that of
the nonvegetarians. In his study of vegetarians, Kirkeby (12)
found only one third as many "fat" individuals among them as
he did among the controls.

That food fiber may be a deterrent to the liability to
overweight is postulated by Heaton (9). He presents three
physiological obstacles to energy intake provided by fiber
in the diet: (1) it displaces calorie-yielding foods, thus
reducing the caloric intake; (2) it requires chewing, which
slows food intake while at the same time producing satiety
by promoting secretion of saliva and gastric juice, which
distends the stomach; (3) it reduces the absorptive efficiency of the small intestine. This reasoning agrees with
the observation of McCance et al. (14) who report that the
fastest eater in their study group took 25 min to eat the
test meal of white bread and 35 min to eat the brown bread
meal. Their slowest eater took 41 min to eat the white bread
and 56 min to down the brown bread. These investigators
found evidence to suggest that the absorption of the white
bread meal was more rapid and complete than that of the brown
bread meal.

D.   Fiber Intake, Blood Pressure, and Serum Cholesterol

In general, we (7) found no significant differences in
blood pressures of the different adult groups. However,
while there were a few hypertensive subjects of approximately
equal numbers among the lacto-ovo-vegetarians and the nonvegetarians, none were found among the pure vegetarians.
Despite their free use of fat, (all-vegetable) the pure
vegetarians had a significantly lower serum cholesterol value
than the nonvegetarians (8). The levels of the lacto-ovo-
vegetarians were intermediate. We observed that an inverse
relationship existed between the fiber content of the diet and
the level of serum cholesterol. The higher the fiber, the
lower the blood cholesterol.

Serum cholesterol levels were higher among our older subjects than among the younger ones. This supports the observation of others that there is a gradual increase in serum cholesterol levels with increasing years. However, this was not the finding of Toomey and White (17) among the Hunzas high in the Himalaya Mountains north of Pakistan. The diet of the Hunzas is spartan and naturally high in fiber. Its mainstay foods are fruits and nuts, vegetables and grains (barley, wheat and millet). Milk is scarce and meat is eaten only once or twice a year on festive occasions. The investigators studied 25 men believed to be 90 to 110 years old. They found normal blood pressures, normal serum cholesterol levels, and normal electrocardiographic patterns. The serum cholesterol values were in the low range of 150 to 180 mg/100 ml.

Kirkeby (12) found some variation of cholesterol values with age in his vegetarian group, but this tendency was less marked than in the controls. The usual sex difference of higher blood cholesterol values in females was present in his vegetarians also, but the characteristic pattern of particularly high levels in women over 50 years of age was not present in his vegetarian subjects.

The church group of vegetarians and nonvegetarians studied by West and Hayes (20) showed the vegetarians to have significantly lower concentrations of cholesterol than the nonvegetarians. Trappist monks on a frugal lacto-vegetarian diet have been reported by Barrow et al. (1), McCullagh and Lewis (15), and Groen et al. (5) to have lower blood cholesterol levels than amnivorous Benedictine monks or men in the general population. Caceres et al. (3), however, report that in spite of the strict adherence of the Trappists to their rigorous regimen, the majority of their study group had serum cholesterol values within, or near, the expected range for the population at large. The authors expressed a lack of evident explanation for this difference between their findings and that of the other researchers.

Trowell (18) calls attention to the suggestion that in Western society the two foods considered effective in reducing hyperlipidemia are the cereal products if taken in large amounts and legumes (peas, beans, peanuts, etc.), all of which have a high fiber content.

Keys et al. (11) failed to find any significant serum
cholesterol-lowering effect whey they added 16 g of cellulose
as a supplement to the diets of middle-aged men, but they did
find a consistent effect from the addition of 15 g of pectin.
The pectin effect was apparent in 3 weeks; it lowered the
serum cholesterol about 5% below the level on the same diet
without the supplement. Pectin is present in most fruits
and berries, particularly in applies and other fruits noted
for the jelly-making properties.

E. Fiber Intake and Colorectal Cancer

The relationship of the fiber intake to the incidence
of colorectal cancer has received much attention in recent
years. Since all our subjects were in apparent good health,
we reported no findings relative to this concern. However,
since most of our adult lacto-ovo-vegetarians were Seventh-
Day Adventists, a 5-year study of Seventh-Day Adventists in
California during the period 1955 to 1959 is of interest (13).
This study found the risk of death from colorectal cancer in
the Adventist population significantly lower than that expected for persons of corresponding age and sex in the
general California population. A continuing study is in
progress. Not all Seventh-Day Adventists are vegetarians,
but those who do eat meat generally consume it only occasionally or in moderate amounts. As has already been pointed
out by ourselves and by West and Hayes, the fiber content of
the diets of this special population group is significantly
greater than that consumed by conventional nonvegetarians.
This higher fiber intake may have had a protective effect
against colorectal cancer.

IV. CONCLUSION

It is generally the case that when the intake of animal
foods is low or entirely lacking, cereal grains and legumes
become the dietary staples of the vegetarian or near-vegetar-
ian diets. Added to these basics are such vegetables and
fruits as the region provides. Thus a vegetarian diet, if
a reasonable selection of foods is available, naturally contains both the high-fiber, cholesterol-lowering seeds (grains
and legumes) together with bulky vegetables, and fruits whose

pectin content tends toward the same end. That this type of
diet is associated with lower serum cholesterol levels than
the diets of omnivorous peoples has been abundantly documented.

REFERENCES

1. Barrow, J. G., Quinlan, C. B., Cooper, G. R., Whitner,
    U. S. and Goodloe, M. R. H., 1960, Studies in athero-
    sclerosis, III. An epidemiologic study of atherosclero-
    sis in Trappist and Benedictine monks. A preliminary
    report, Ann. Int. Med., 52:368.

2. Burkitt, D. P., Walker, A. R. P. and Painter, N. S.,
    1974, Dietary fiber and disease, J. A. M. A., 229:1068.

3. Caceres, C. A., Calatayud, J. B., Orvis, H. H., Fawal,
    I. A., Thomas, R., Kelser, G. A., Abraham, S. and
    Anderson, A., 1963, An evaluation of clinical and
    laboratory findings in male subjects on long-term,
    low-fat, low-protein diets, New Engl. J. Med., 269:550.

4. Cowgill, G. R. and Anderson, W. E., 1932, Laxative
    effects of wheat bran and "washed bran" in healthy men.
    A comparative study, J. A. M. A., 98:1866.

5. Groein, J. J., Tijong, K. B., Koster, M., Willebrands,
    A. F., Verdonck, G. and Pierloot, M., 1962, The influ-
    ence of nutrition and ways of life on blood cholesterol
    and the prevalence of hypertension and coronary heart
    disease among Trappist and Benedictine monks, Am. J.
    Clin. Nutr., 10:456.

6. Hardinge, M. G., Chambers, A. C. and Crooks, H., 1958,
    Nutritional studies of vegetarians, III. Dietary
    levels of fiber, Amer. J. Clin, Nutr., 6:523.

7. Hardinge, M. G. and Stare, F. J., 1954, Nutritional
    studies of vegetarians, I. Nutritional, physical, and
    laboratory studies, J. Clin, Nutr., 23:73.

8. Hardinge, M. G. and Stare, F. J., 1954, Nutritional
    studies of vegetarians, II. Dietary and serum levels
    of cholesterol, J. Clin. Nutr., 2:83.

9. Heaton, K. W., 1973, Food fiber as an obstacle to energy intake, Lancet, 2:1418.

10. Hindhede, M., 1920, The effect of food restriction during war on mortality in Copenhagen, J. A. M. A., 74:381.

11. Keys, A., Grande, F. and Anderson, J. T., 1961, Fiber and pectin in the diet and serum cholesterol concentration in man, Proc. Soc. Experl. Biol. Med., 106:555.

12. Kirkeby, K., 1966, Blood lipids, lipoproteins, and proteins in vegetarians, Acta Med. Scandinav., 179 Suppl., 443:59.

13. Lemon, F. R., Walden, R. T. and Woods, R. W., 1964, Cancer of the lung and mouth in Seventh-Day Adventists. A preliminary report on a population study, Cancer, 17:486.

14. McCance, R. A., Prior, K. M. and Painter, N. S., 1953, A radiological study of the rate of passage of brown and white bread through the digestive tract of man, Brit. J. Nutr., 7:98.

15. McCullagh, E. P. and Lewis, L. A., 1960, A study of diet, blood lipids and vascular disease in Trappist monks, New Engl. J. Med., 263:569.

16. Payler, D. K., 1973, Food fiber and bowel behavior, Lancet, 1:1394.

17. Toomey, E. G. and White, P. D., 1964, A brief survey of the health of aged Hunzas, Am. Heart J., 68:841.

18. Trowell, H., 1972, Ischemic heart disease and dietary fiber, Am. J. Clin. Nutr., 25:926.

19. Watt, B. K. and Merrill, A. L., 1950, Composition of foods - raw, processed, prepared, U. S. D. A. Handbook No. 8.

20. West, R. O. and Hayes, O. B., 1968, Diet and serum cholesterol levels: A comparison between vegetarians and nonvegetarians in a Seventh-Day Adventist group, Amer. J. Clin. Nutr., 21:853.

CHAPTER 6

FERMENTATION AS THE PRINCIPAL CAUSE

OF THE PHYSIOLOGICAL ACTIVITY OF INDIGESTIBLE FOOD RESIDUE

Emile W. Hellendoorn

Central Institute for Nutrition
and Food Research

Zeist, The Netherlands

I.   INTRODUCTION

The vegetable kingdom is not only the object of research for the botanist, it also supplies the basic materials for the paper and textile industries, and provides food for animals and man. Since the research aspects differ, investigators in the various disciplines approach the plant each from his own field of activity.

Nutritionists only recently became interested in the physiological aspects of plant cell wall constituents in human nutrition. They had been greatly influenced by the knowledge about fiber gathered by chemists working with wood and cellulose and by animal nutritionists who had accumulated a fund of information on the digestibility of forage plants and developed an analytical approach to the study. However, human vegetable foods are not as lignified as wood and not as fibrous and cellulosic as forage plants. Human food consists of many parts of the plant which, on chewing, readily lose their structure, and rough, fibrous, stringy, or tough parts are discarded during preparation or spit out before being swallowed.

Therefore, the terms "roughage," "fiber" and, particularly, "cellulose," are not applicable to the indigestible parts of vegetable human food and should no longer be used in this context.

The use of the term "rough" as a contrast to "smooth"
when referring to food components (58) is also misleading;
it strengthens the misconception that such rough parts irri-
tate the inner wall of the human digestive tract mechani-
cally. The modern conception is that fiber does not irri-
tate the gut (2). For example, bran may be hard and rough
when dry, but it becomes smooth after adequate imbibition
of water or saliva, just as does other dry or dehydrated
vegetable material.

Whether they originate in the cell wall or in the cell
content, the indigestible components of food plants are,
as a group, of greater significance in the physiology of
nutrition than those parts defined only as "fiber." It is
more appropriate to think in terms of the soluble and the
insoluble indigestible components of human food (Table 1).

In human food plants, the hemicellulose portion domi-
nates; the cellulose and lignin content is small compared
to that in forage plants. In respect to constitution, pectin may be considered part of the complex hemicellulose
group. However, the older concept that hemicelluloses are
distinctively insoluble in water and soluble in dilute alkaline solutions is still supported (Figure 1).

TABLE 1. Indigestible Components of Vegetable Foods

Insoluble components (called fiber, bulk, roughage or "cellulose")	Soluble components
Cellulose (slightly fermentable)	Pectin (readily fermentable)
Hemicellulose (mostly fermentable)	Galacto-oligosaccharides (readily fermentable)
Lignin (not fermentable)	

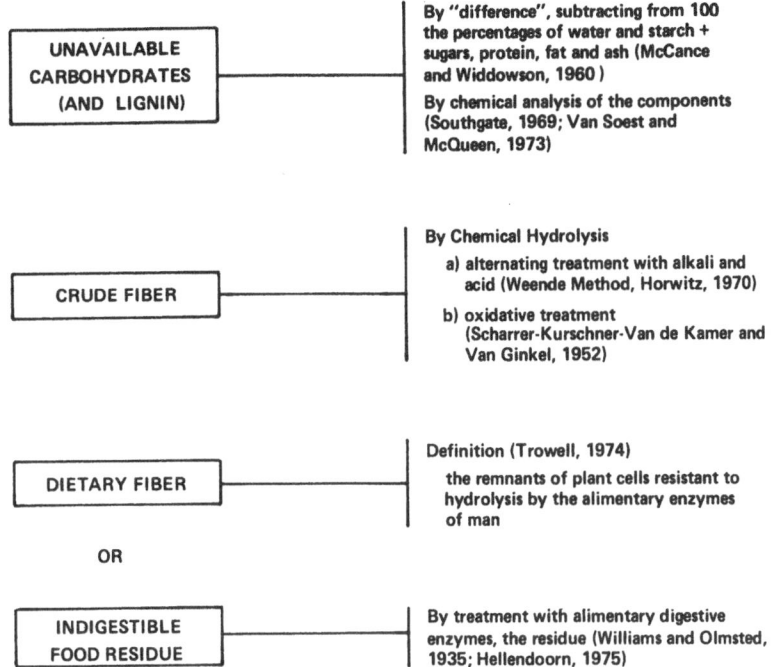

Figure 1. Classification of the hemicellulose group after Norman (49).

Trowell postulated a physiological concept of fiber, which he called dietary fiber and defined as the remnants of plant cells that are not hydrolyzed by the alimentary enzymes of man (65). As was mentioned previously, some objections exist to the use of the term "fiber" at all, because this term is too closely associated with the botanical concept of fiber, even in such expressions as "dietary fiber" and especially "plant fiber" (57), since we are concerned only with plant material anyway. We prefer to use the term "indigestible residue" after Williams and Olmsted (73), a term that clearly reflects what is actually going on in the small intestine.

The method for determining in vitro the indigestible part of vegetable human food (Figure 2) must match as closely as possible the physiological concept of the indigestible residue (dietary fiber ∿ unavailable carbohydrates + lignin).

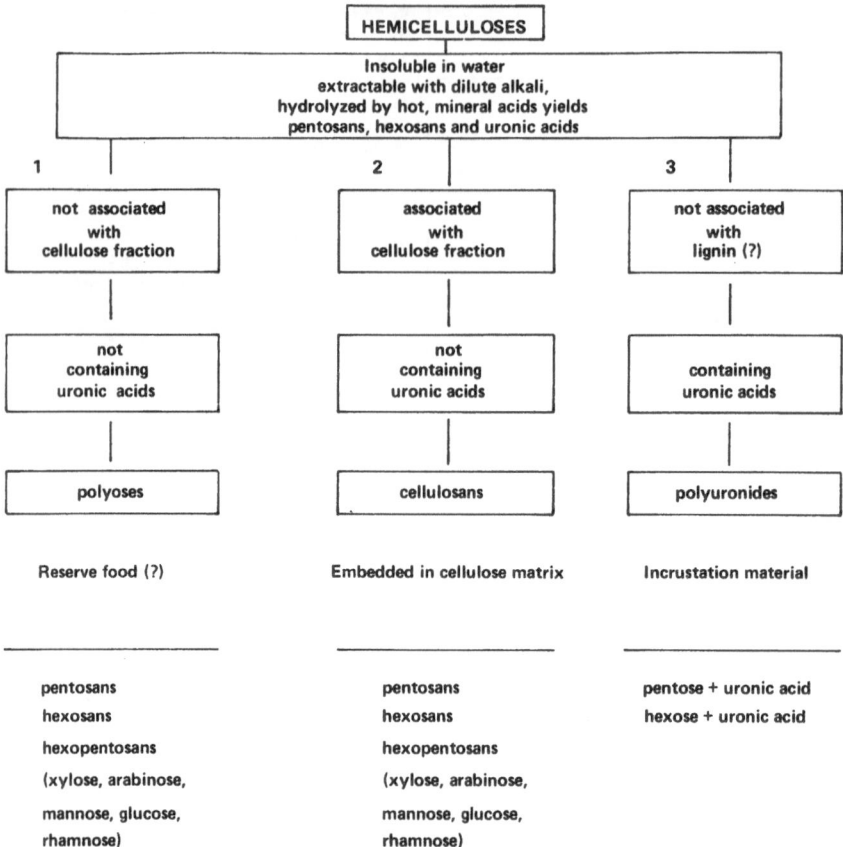

Figure 2.   Methods for the determination of the indigestible part of human vegetable food.

Therefore, chemical analytical methods are unsuitable; enzymatic methods that make use of enzymes from micro-organisms are generally not reliable, as it is unlikely that these enzymes will hydrolyze the carbohydrates according to exactly the same pattern of attack as the digestive enzymes do. The risk is undoubtedly present that they continue to degrade the undigested polysaccharides, so that hydrolysis progresses to the extent that is normally the hydrolyzing function of the colon bacteria.

II. THE INDIGESTIBLE RESIDUE OF VEGETABLE FOODS AND ITS FATE IN THE BODY

For determination of the indigestible residue (IR) content of human vegetable foods, an enzymatic method has been developed which uses pepsin and pancreatin in the presence of sodium dodecyl (lauryl) sulfate as the surface active agent (24).

The results of determinations of the IR content of some vegetable foods, along with their crude fiber (CF) content, are given in Table 2. As the water content of the various foods varies widely, CF values and IR values are given as percentages of dry matter.

Discrepancies between CF and IR are considerable with leguminous seeds and with whole-wheat products. Among legumes, peanuts and soyflour, which were defatted previously, have lower IR values than peas and beans. During tempeh[1] fermentation, part of the indigestible matter has disappeared. The IR content of peas and beans is comparable with that of whole-wheat and rye products, the latter having the highest value. The lowest IR values are found with white bread and polished rice. Rolled oats has an intermediate IR content.

IR values of most vegetables are very high, as are their CF values. The high percentages of CF in respect to IR show that most vegetables are more "cellulosic" than beans and cereals. In the natural state, the high water content more or less "dilutes" the indigestible matter of vegetables, and thus their contribution to the indigestible matter in the daily diet is not as high as the IR values suggest. However, cassava leaves, one third of which is indigestible, are consumed in great quantities by the Papuas of New Guinea.

IR values of vegetables do not change significantly on cooking (24). Therefore, cooking does not imply a chemical breakdown of the indigestible components; the reported improved digestibility of vegetables on cooking must therefore be caused by easier accessibility to components by digestive juices, probably generated by hydrogen-bond breaking.

---

[1] Indonesian fermented soybean product.

TABLE 2.   Comparison of Crude Fiber Content (Weende Method)
            and Indigestible Residue Content
            (Enzymatic Method) of Various Foods

Food product	Dry matter content of product (%)	Crude Fiber (%)	Indigestible residue(%)
		(dry weight basis)	
Legumes			
Kidney beans, pressure cooked	80.5	2.8	15.0
White beans ⎫	29.9	2.3	15.7
Dun peas ⎬ canned	26.2	2.3	19.6
Peas ⎭	24.9	2.3	13.2
Soybeans	92.7	2.4	5.1
Soyflour (defatted)	88.1	7.5	11.9
Tempeh[1]	49.8	6.0	6.8
Peanuts (defatted)	96.5	2.6	8.0
Cereal products			
Rolled oats	89.4	1.7	7.7
Rice (polished)	86.5	0.7	1.6
White bread	56.2	0.8	4.0
Whole-wheat bread	59.6	2.0	15.5
Rye bread	66.2	1.6	21.0
Wheat bran	87.1	10.4	56.0
Fruits			
Apples	16.4	∿4	∿7
Pears	13.6	∿10	∿8
Vegetables			
Potatoes	20.7	2.8	9.9
Endive ⎫	94.2	13.0	21.7
Curled kale ⎪	92.0	9.0	30.2
Cassava leaves ⎬ Dehy-	95.8	10.5	34.6
White cabbage ⎪ drated	88.6	17.5	21.5
Carrots ⎪	89.3	9.0	9.9
Onions ⎭	94.1	10.0	10.5

Source: Hellendoorn, 1975.
[1]Indonesian fermented soybean product.

The IR value found through determination represents the insoluble part of the indigestible plant material: cellulose, hemicellulose, lignin, protopectin, and some indigestible proteinous material such as extensine. Individual components of IR may be determined according to the scheme given by Southgate (55). However, one should bear in mind that IR is not merely the sum of the separated components, as association, or physical bonding, and incrustation greatly influence enzymatic degradability. Soluble pectin may be determined as monogalacturonic acid in the combined filtrate and washings, using the carbazole sulfuric acid reagent (68); a simple method for determination of galacto-oligosaccharides as a group or separately is not yet available (35). The method may also be applied to food of animal origin, resulting in a residue of collagenous indigestible proteins.

According to the procedure, enzymatic hydrolysis of the food product is carried out to such an extent that digestion is optimal. With natural food products, no distinct limit does in fact exist between digestible and indigestible carbohydrates; on the contrary, some fluctuations may be found according to the activity of the enzymatic treatment.

In-vivo digestion of normally digestible carbohydrates of food may not go as far as in the case of the in-vitro determination, if the organism is lacking in digestive capacity relative to the supply of carbohydrates. This failure may be caused by the food product itself, when parts of the carbohydrates are less accessible or more resistant to hydrolysis; it may be caused, too, by a deficiency in hydrolyzing capacity of the individual organism itself, a deficiency that may be hereditary or only temporary. It may also be the result of insufficient reaction time to digest and absorb properly as with the short-small-bowel syndrome, or the result of a too-rapid food transit. In all these situations, digestible unabsorbed carbohydrates are liable to attack by micro-organisms of the lower intestine; they increase the effect of fermentation of the indigestible carbohydrates of the food.

As will be seen in Table 2, with most food products the IR values, the residue remaining after enzymatic hydrolysis, largely exceed CF values, the residue remaining after chemical hydrolysis. This shows that, with CF determination, only a smaller fraction of fiber resists chemical hydrolysis. In the future, neutral detergent fiber will possibly be substituted for CF (69).

According to the present author, the favorable as well as the undesirable physiological action of the undigested residue may largely be ascribed to fermentation of the fermentable part of the undigested residue in the large intestine (22).

Analysis of the feces for the presence of fiber material has shown (56, 74, 75) that the greater part of the cellulose and lignin of the food ingested can be recovered in the stool. The major part of hemicelluloses, however, are fermented in the large intestine; only smaller parts can be found in the stool (Table 1).

By gross approximation, we may take CF as a measure for the nonfermentable part of IR. Or, which is the same thing:

$$\text{IR minus CF} \sim \text{fermentable part of IR}$$

In addition to the fermentation of this part of the insoluble undigested residue, soluble pectin and the galacto-oligosaccharides are also fermented (Table 1), as are part of the carbohydrates, those which are normally digested and absorbed in the small intestine but have escaped complete absorption. These include some starches that are difficult to digest, and disaccharides in the case of disaccharidase-deficient people.

Some workers still take the results of feces analysis as a measure for carbohydrate digestibility, as with the digestibility of protein and fat. They ignore the fact that those carbohydrates escaping hydrolysis by the alimentary enzymes and absorption in the small intestine are fermented to a greater or lesser extent by the enzymes of the colon bacteria and thus are nearly totally calorically unavailable. In addition to the fermentation in the colon of non-absorbed exogenous carbohydrates, fermentation of endogenous mucus-polysaccharides has to be taken into account (72).

Fermentation of the unabsorbed food carbohydrates gives rise to different end products with different physiological effects, as shown schematically in Figure 3.

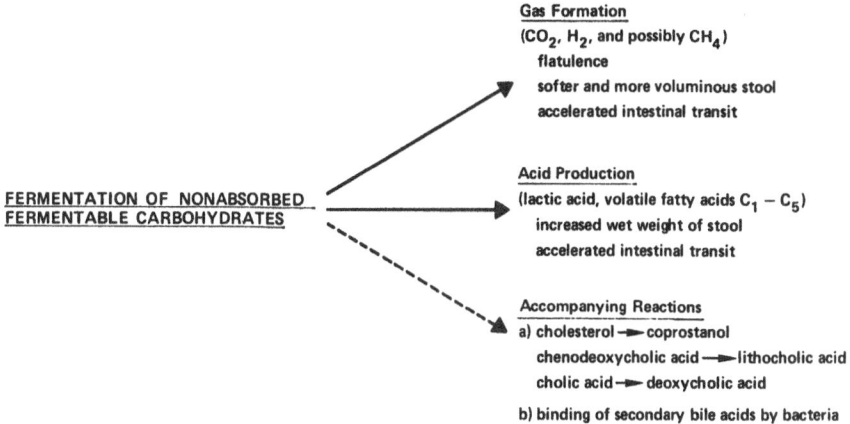

Figure 3.   Fermentation of the fermentable part of the undigested residue of vegetable foods.

Of course, the expression "fermentation of carbohydrates" (carbohydrates normally dominate in such a complex system as that represented by the food residue in the lumen of the intestine) is here used in a wider sense; it is not limited to gas formation and acid production but denotes all normal microbial activity in which lipids are also involved. The abnormal condition of putrefaction of proteins (that has become almost normal for people in the West) is excluded.

People's fermentative reactions are, however, highly individual. Each subject has his own distinctive pattern of intestinal microbial flora; eating habits also differ from one subject to another. Obviously, it is difficult to decide whether a subject's reaction should be called normal or abnormal. Moreover, a person's reaction should not be regarded as a constant datum; it may fluctuate in intensity and in end products for short or long periods of time.

By the enzymatic procedure, sufficient quantities of IR of food products may be isolated and then freeze-dried for the study of the physiological effects in experiments with animals and man.

III.   VARIABLE RATE OF STARCH DIGESTION

The starch content of foods can be determined in several analytical ways, chemical as well as enzymatic methods can be used and may yield different results (63). Therefore, no exact analytical characterization of starch can be given; nor is it possible to give an exact physiological characterization of starch, as digestion may not always be completed.

On chemical or microscopical examination of the stool, only small amounts of the starch of the food consumed can be recovered (19, 56). This is, however, not an indication of nearly complete digestibility of starch, as unabsorbed starch has largely been fermented in the large intestine and is, as such, no longer detectable in the stool.

It is well known that the starch of bread becomes, on staling, less easy to digest in vitro by salivary or pancreatic amylolytic enzymes (30, 32). The diminished rate of hydrolysis by digestive enzymes of the starch of stale bread and of insufficiently baked bread could be correlated with the blood sugar curves of humans after ingestion of these sorts of bread; by this means both digestion and absorption in the small intestine could be measured (39). Usually, however, in normal eating practice the diminished digestibility of stale bread is not observed, as stale white bread is masticated and mixed with saliva more thoroughly than fresh bread, which is softer. This phenomenon can be demonstrated by X-ray examination of the chewing effect: fresh bread is badly chewed and remains in the form of distinct lumps in the stomach for long periods of time. Old bread is chewed into more finely divided particles, which are more easily accessible to hydrolysis by digestive enzymes (41, 64).

Williams and Olmsted observed that a diet rich in carbohydrates--even in such an easily digestible form as wheat starch--increases the bulk of the stool more than does a diet rich in protein or fat (74, 75).

In-vitro digestibility measurements of dehydrated mashed potato products show that the rate of digestion of the granular products is inferior to that of the flakes. This difference in digestibility between the two products is caused by the physical phenomenon of hardening, or retrograda-

tion, of the potato starch during manufacture of the granules, adversely affecting digestibility. Under certain
physiological conditions, potato granules, when consumed
in large quantities, may cause such minor digestive discom-
forts as intestinal gas and a puffed feeling (20, 26).

Various starches differ in their digestibility (52).
Raw starches of potatoes and dry beans give rise to diarrhea
and flatulence. Thus the digestibility of these kinds of
starch depends on cooking time. As a dietetic measure, only
potato flakes or well-cooked potatoes should be given to
patients with digestive troubles. Some 5 to 10% of the
starch of beans of good cooking quality remains difficult
to digest.

Our investigations showed that dry beans harvested
the previous year and kept under unfavorable conditions of
temperature and humidity have bad cooking qualities. Of
the starch of such beans, 10 to 15% remains indigestible
even after prolonged cooking (19). Before doing these in-
vitro digestibility measurements, we determined the total
amount of starch present in the beans by treating them with
cold 4 N hydrochloric acid to make the starch available for
amylolysis. The indigestible part of the starch of such
beans, although still referred to as starch, has physiologically been added to the amount of indigestible components
of the cell wall.

IV.   FERMENTATION AS THE CAUSE OF INTESTINAL GAS FORMATION

Research on gas-forming properties of foods, stimulated
by NASA, had as its object the elucidation of the cause of
flatulence and the escape of gas by the rectum. Dry beans
having been reported to be notorious gas-formers (45), investigations centered on subjects after they had consumed
meals including beans.

Among investigators the view prevailed that some
"flatulence-active principle," some chemically stimulating
agent, would be responsible for gas formation and that this
component should be discovered.

The principal results of the investigations of the American research teams will be only briefly reviewed here (5, 21,
38).

Rectal gas consists of carbon dioxide, hydrogen, and often methane. The volume of gas produced, as well as the relative amounts of the constituent gases, are highly individual; some people produce methane; others do not (46).

Originally, some agent present in beans was thought to stimulate the secretion of pancreatic juice, resulting in the evolution of carbon dioxide gas from the bicarbonate present (59). Later Steggerda and coworkers concluded from their experiments with animals and human subjects, in which a mixture of antimicrobial drugs was used, that gas production by beans could be largely inhibited. This result is only compatible with the view that gas production in the gut is a microbial process (60).

The technique by which hydrogen gas in the breath is measured replaced the necessity for measuring rectal gas; this technique much stimulated research. Peak gas production occurs about 6 hr after consumption of a meal of beans. This coincides with the time necessary for the food to reach the ileocecal region, the food still being in the small intestine (8, 45). Levitt, however, was of the opinion that gas production in great quantities has to take place in the cecum and not in the ileum, as the microbial population of the small intestine would be too small for that function: 10^2 to 10^5 organisms/ml vs 10^{10} to 10^{11}/ml in the colon (38). The cause of rapid gas production and flatulence in some people, reported to start even within half an hour after ingestion of meals and coming to an end far within 6 hr, has probably to be sought in the intestinal reflex, expelling gas that is still present in the intestine and that was already formed after ingestion of the previous meal.

Production of hydrogen gas may not have the same cause as production of carbon dioxide. Experiments with certain antimicrobial drugs indicate that these two gases have different origins; for example, the hydrogen component of flatus was more reduced than the carbon dioxide component (46).

Murphy attempted to isolate and identify the gas-producing factor of dry beans by successive physical and chemical treatment, then tested each successive fraction by feeding it to human subjects and measuring the resulting breath and flatus gas. He found that the factor is

TABLE 3. Flatus-producing Influence of Some Food Products
          in One Ambulant Human Test Subject

Test food	Quantity of intake (dry matter in g)	Flatus production (ml/24h)	Avg increase in flatus volume (ml/100g dry product)
Normal diet (18x)		235 $\pm$ 15	
Kidney beans	250/175/160	1730/1220/960	540
Dun peas	125/210/210	500/1160/930	330
Lentils	200/200	990/820	335
Green peas	200	800	280
Kidney beans + onions + parsley	125	1250	810
Dutch onions	95/80	900/1400	1080
Italian onions	115	4340	3500
Egyptian onions	105	2430	2100

Source: Hellendoorn, 1969.

extractable with 60% aqueous ethanol, and thus has to be
sought in the low-molecular-weight components. Attention
focused on the soluble galacto-oligosaccharides raffinose and
stachyose (sugars built up, respectively, of one galactose
and one sucrose unit and two galactose units and one sucrose
unit) present in the active fraction. These sugars are not
hydrolyzed and not absorbed in the small intestine. They
thus form a substrate for microbial fermentation in lower
parts of the gut (9, 48).

    Most investigators agree that the flatulence-active fac-
tor of beans must be sought in the soluble low-molecular-
weight carbohydrate components and not in the high-molecular-
weight fraction. This especially applies to the hydrogen
component of flatus, but whether this is also true of the
carbon dioxide component is not quite certain. The question
arises as to the possible fate of these indigestible high-
molecular-weight components of beans in the intestine.

    With one ambulant human test subject who reacted on his
normal diet with a fairly constant flatus volume over the day,
we measured the relative activity of different legumes and
onions (Table 3) (19). Some difference in flatus-forming ac-

tivity was found among different leguminous seeds. Onions produced an enormous flatus volume. However, the quantities which were consumed were far in excess of normal. Nevertheless, the flatulence activity of onions, on dry-weight bases, is much greater than that of beans.

In another experiment with two human ambulant test subjects, the share of the cuticle in flatulence activity of kidney beans was measured. Flatus gas was measured over the whole day, when, respectively, on a diet with whole beans, deskinned beans (93% on dry-weight basis), and the skins only (7% on dry-weight basis) (Table 4). In both subjects, whole beans as well as the cotyledons exerted about the same effect on flatulence. The cuticles, however, had only a minor effect, corresponding with their share in the total crude fiber content of the beans, about 15%. Consequently, the flatulence-stimulating effect of whole beans cannot be attributed to the skins of the beans. This result appeared to be in agreement with the results of the experiments on transit of the food in rats, when the skins only slightly accelerated transit.

In experiments with rats (10 animals in each experiment), cooked beans were substituted for wheat starch in their rations. An increase in intestinal gas volume of 25 to 30% could be observed 6 hr after feeding. This increase in gas volume remained even after prolonged cooking or retorting of the beans. The intestinal gas volume measured was approximately the same for soft-cooking as for hard-cooking beans, the differences in digestibility of the bean starch being too small to influence the results (19).

To investigate the possible existence of a flatulence-active component of beans, we extracted dehydrated cooked beans with 60% alcohol. In three experiments with rats, rations with the extracted beans and with the extracts were compared with the basal ration (Table 5). A distinct rise in gas volume resulted from the intake of cooked whole beans. Although the extracted beans produced gas volumes that remained below the values obtained with whole beans, the effects were still appreciable. The extracts showed only a minor activity compared to the activity of nonextracted beans. In an experiment with rats using an extraction of beans, a similar result was obtained with intestinal transit. (See Table 8.)

TABLE 4. Flatus Volume of Two Ambulant Test Subjects on a Diet With Whole Beans, Deskinned Beans, and Bean Skins

Test food		Subject A (200 g dry beans)		Subject B (150 g dry beans)	
		Flatus (ml/24h)	Increase in flatus (ml/100g)	Flatus (ml/24h)	Increase in flatus (ml/100g)
Basal (without beans)	(5x)	220 ± 80	-	118 ± 7	-
Whole beans	(2x)	780 ± 160	280	368 ± 48	167
Deskinned beans[1]	(2x)	725 ± 95	253	375 ± 55	173
Bean skins[2]	(2x)	265 ± 15	23	140 ± 10	15

Source: Hellendoorn, 1969.

[1] 93% on dry-weight basis.

[2] 7% on dry-weight basis.

TABLE 5. Intestinal Gas Volume of Rats
on a Basal Ration, and on Rations
with Whole Beans, Extracted Beans, and Bean Extract

Ration	Average intestinal gas volume (ml)		
	Expt. 1	Expt. 2	Expt. 3
Basal (without beans)	1.02 ± 0.18	1.02 ± 0.18	1.02 ± 0.18
Whole beans	1.91 ± 0.21	2.49 ± 0.14	2.28 ± 0.15
Extracted beans	1.73 ± 0.16	2.25 ± 0.16	2.20 ± 0.09
Bean extract	1.20 ± 0.15	1.47 ± 0.17	1.45 ± 0.08

Source: Hellendoorn, 1969.

Measuring flatus volume in three ambulant human subjects, we found the effect of alcoholic extraction to be less clear (Table 6). Extracted beans showed a minor activity in test subjects A and C; test subject B reacted to extracted beans with a response comparable to flatulence formation with the intake of whole beans. The extracts themselves showed no activity. Thus, from our experiments we may conclude that the majority of the flatulence-active components of beans are not extractable with aqueous alcohol; most of the activity must be sought in the nonextractable high-molecular-weight bean fraction.

As shown by the experiments with human subjects, some flatulence always occurs, even after intake of a diet low in residue content, the greater part originating from swallowed air, the minor part from intestinal gas production.

To prove the hypothesis that intestinal gas production is the result of fermentation, we tried to measure an increase in acid production by analyzing the feces of test subjects on a bean diet for lactic acid and the volatile fatty acids, as production of these acids always accompanies fermentation of carbohydrates (71). We failed to detect a significant increase in acid content of the feces in our first experiments with rats, since not only do rats produce these acids in their large cecum by fermentation, but absorption makes the acids calorically available to a large degree.

With humans, however, these acids are only slowly absorbed
and the majority is excreted with the feces.

A variable increase in lactic acid, formic acid, acetic
acid, propionic acid, and isobutyric or butyric acid could
be detected in the stools of four human test subjects who
were consuming beans daily (150 g on dry-weight basis) during a whole week. (See Table 9.) These acid fermentation
products decrease pH of feces; pH tends to be increased when
some putrefaction of protein takes place simultaneously.

The reverse may be even more important. In contrast
to the normal neutral pH of Western stools, the feces of
Ugandans living on a high-residue, low-protein diet is normally acid (pH 5 to 6); the result is that they very rarely
carry Cl. paraputrificans in their guts (27).

The lowest pH found in this experiment of the stools of
subjects while on an intake of beans was 5.9. At this and
lower pH values of the stool, some carbon dioxide is released
from the bicarbonate originating in the pancreatic fluid excreted during digestion; this additional CO_2 formation is the
indirect result of the primary fermentative acid formation in
the lower intestine.

TABLE 6. Flatulence Activity of Beans, Extracted Beans,
and the Bean Extracts in Three Human Test Subjects

Test food	Flatus volume in ml/24h per 100 g of dry beans		
	Subject A	Subject B	Subject C
Basal (with-out beans)	200 ± 40 (6x)	130 ± 20 (8x)	<50 (5x)
Brown beans	300/430	255/310	–
Extracted beans	250/215	185/300/370	50/90
Bean extract	200 ± 40 (2x)	130 ± 20 (3x)	<50 (2x)

Source: Hellendoorn, 1969.

Starch content of the stools in the bean-diet period
was not significantly increased; thus the less-digestible,
nonabsorbed part of bean starch (about 5 to 10% of dry beans)
is fermented in the large intestine.

Originally, our ad hoc hypothesis was that this nonabsorbed part of starch was the only agent responsible for
fermentative gas formation. Later we came to the conclusion
that the total amount of indigestible carbohydrates of beans
far exceeds the percentage of less-digestible starch.

By calculating the unavailable part of beans, including
lignin, a value of 12 to 15% on dry-weight basis was obtained,
to which 5% less-digestible bean starch may be added.

Crude-fiber values of the stools did not reflect crude-
fiber values of the beans ingested, some being higher and
some being lower; more data would be necessary to draw conclusions.

At the time we were doing these experiments (1965-1966),
no clear definitions existed for the terms fiber, crude
fiber, unavailable carbohydrates, and indigestible part of
the food; there were no direct, analytical methods except
for crude fiber. These circumstances led to the development
of an enzymatic method for the determination of the IR content of beans (21), followed by an improved procedure by
which filtration was simplified and speeded up (24).

Experiments must still be done to determine what part
of the IR content of ingested food leaves the intestine unfermented by analyzing the intake and the stool by the enzymatic method. Data from the literature indicate that a substantial amount of fiber is lost by fermentation (56, 74, 75).
As is mentioned in Section II, CF will be regarded approximately as the final residue of the indigestible part of the
food after digestion and fermentation have taken place, and
IR minus CF as the fermentable part of IR. However, chemical
and bacterial degradation of fiber are, of course, not iden-
tical; lignin, for example, is not hydrolyzed by bacterial
enzymes, but is hydrolyzed to a large extent during the more
drastic chemical crude-fiber determination.

Considering CF values and IR values of various foods
(Table 2), the differences between the two are greatest
with leguminous seeds and whole-wheat products. A fairly

consistent relation can be observed between the magnitude
of this difference and reported flatulence activity. Beans
and dun peas are more flatulent than soybeans, tempeh,
or peanuts; rye bread and whole-wheat bread are more flatulent than rolled oats and the refined cereals; potatoes are
flatulent when consumed in appreciable amounts.

With vegetables, CF values are relatively higher and
correlations with gas-forming properties are less clear.
In the analyzed sample of dehydrated onions, no difference
at all was found between CF and IR value; yet onions are
highly flatulent (Table 4). By analysis of onions dehydrated
in the laboratory, an IR content of 6.0% and a CF value of
2.7% were found, a difference still too small to explain
flatulence activity. Soluble pectin, determined in the filtrate, amounted to only 2.9%. The observation that onions
are practically nonflatulent when consumed as such after
fasting but exhibit their activity only when consumed in combination with starchy foods, as is most normal, may lead to
the tentative explanation that onions contain a component
pharmacodynamically stimulating peristalsis, so that starch
rather than onions is in reality the substrate for fermentation.

Of course, no strict relation may ever be found between
IR and CF and fermentative reactivity. Not only may the
soluble indigestible components have a dominating influence
with some foods, for example fruits and vegetables, but
qualitative differences in the composition of IR may deter
mine the course of fermentation, producing various gases and
acids as fermentation metabolites in variable amounts.

Intestinal gas formation should not be considered entirely undesirable. Gas entrapped in the moving fecal mass
gives it a softer consistency and increases the volume,
greatly facilitating its propulsion. This aspect of fermentation is incorporated in the experiments on transit time
dealt with in Section V.

               V.   FERMENTATION AS THE CAUSE OF ACCELERATED
                        TRANSIT IN THE LARGE BOWEL

Accelerated bowel transit is observed in persons who
follow traditional habits of eating natural, unrefined foods
high in fiber (6). One could better say that their bowel

transit is normal, and that the bowel transit of people in
the West with a low fiber intake is delayed. In addition
to accelerated transit, these people have to eliminate their
food debris more frequently than people in the West, and
their stools are more voluminous and softer.

However, the authors who made these observations fail
to explain how fiber decreases transit time and how exactly
it contributes to a more voluminous and softer stool. The
view is often encountered that these phenomena have a purely
physical cause, starting with water binding by fiber (13).
We will show, however, that the primary cause must be sought
in bacterial action in the bowel resulting in acid production
that accompanies gas formation.

In our experiments, carried out at the Institute in
1965 and 1966 to investigate the cause of the gas-forming
properties of beans (see Section IV), we observed an increase
in the rate of transit through the bowel of rats, which were
taught to obtain only one short-time meal a day, when part of
the starch in their diet was replaced by beans. We carried
out the tests for each ration with 10 individually housed
rats and averaged the values obtained. (Table 7.) The feces
of rats whose diet contained 15 or 30% of beans, respectively, was transported more quickly through the intestine than
was that of rats on the control diet that contained wheat
starch.

Figures on bowel transit time for the animals whose
diet contained raw beans or beans that had only been heated
to boiling are not fully comparable with those of the rats
on the rations with cooked beans, because the former groups
developed serious diarrhea and consumed far less food than
did the latter. This proved that the antinutritional factors
of the beans were only destroyed by cooking.

The rate of transit was highest with beans cooked for
only 5 min and given in the higher concentration of 30% of
the ration. A distinct acceleration of transit, 20 to 25%,
was observed even after prolonged cooking or after retorting.

The results of these experiments can be related to the
in-vitro digestibility of beans when cooked for varying
times. The raw beans contained 48% starch. The starch content was determined by pretreating the beans with cold 4 N

TABLE 7. Bowel Transit Times in Rats while on Rations with Beans

| Rations | Average bowel transit times | | | |
| | 30% beans | | 15% beans | |
	(min)	(%)	(min)	(%)
Unheated	260	86	270	81
Beans heated to boiling	271	90	284	85
Beans cooked for 5 min	211	70	249	75
Beans cooked for 10 min	222	73	249	75
Beans cooked for 30 min	233	77	250	75
Beans cooked for 60 min	232	77	255	76
Beans retorted at 120°C for 120 min	251	83	266	80
Basal (without beans)	303	100	325	100

Source: Hellendoorn, 1969.

Note: All beans were of good cooking quality and were soaked overnight.

hydrochloric acid to make the starch susceptible to amylolysis. The starch of the raw beans, which had been soaked
overnight, was only about 20% digested. Digestibility
appeared to increase rapidly upon cooking, so that after
1 hr normal cooking the starch was 85% digestible, and
after pressure cooking, about 90%. The calculated total
carbohydrate content of the raw beans amounts to about 60
to 63%, which exceeds the starch content by 12 to 15%.
These nonstarch carbohydrates are unavailable and, added
to the 5% indigestible starch, make a total of nearly 20%
of the beans. This figure is in agreement with the data
found by direct in-vitro determination (Table 2).

The increase in starch digestibility on cooking is
reflected in a decrease in transit time. The influence
of the indigestible portion of fully cooked beans is reflected in the 25 to 30% increase in transit time, which
remains after prolonged cooking.

Beans of poor cooking quality did not reach a higher
digestibility than about 85% after prolonged cooking or
retorting. However, the difference in digestibility from
that of the soft-cooking beans was too small to be reflected
in the experiments on transit time.

Another experiment, in which wheat starch was replaced
by an equivalent amount of beans, deskinned beans, and the
skins themselves, respectively, indicated that the accelerating influence of beans on the bowel transit time of rats
is caused mainly by the cotyledons of the beans and only to
a minor degree by the cuticles.

In two experiments, rations with extracted beans, which
after normal cooking were dehydrated, ground to a powder,
and then extracted twice with 60% alcohol during 2 hr under
reflux and with the extracts, respectively, were compared
with the basal ration. Effects on transit time are given
in Table 8. When comparing the transit time of rats on
rations containing the extract, no decrease was observed
for that of those on the control ration.

Acceleration of bowel transit, however, occurs with
rations containing respectively 30 and 40% of extracted
beans. Consequently, acceleration of bowel transit of rats

TABLE 8. Bowel Transit Time in Rats on the Basal Ration,
on a Ration with Extracted Beans, and on a
Ration with Bean Extract

Ration	Transit time	
	(min)	(%)
Experiment I		
Basal (without beans)	258	100
Ration with extracted beans (30%)	200	81
Ration with bean extract	265	103
Experiment II		
Basal (without beans)	314	100
Ration with extracted beans (40%)	239	76
Ration with bean extract	312	99

Source: Hellendoorn, 1969.

is not caused by some factor present in beans that stimulates
peristalsis and is extractable with aqueous alcohol.

The cause must be sought in fermentation in the intestine of the nonassimilated carbohydrates and in the formation of acids and gases. In this context, the formation of
acids is of primary interest.

In experiments with four human subjects consuming beans
during one week, an increase in acid content of their stools
was observed. The bean-diet period was preceded by a 7-day
control period during which the experimental subjects consumed fixed quantities, but varying from subject to subject,
of food products with low fiber content. In the bean-diet
period, 150 g of beans (dry-weight basis) were consumed
daily, the calories of bread and potatoes were reduced, but
the other meal components were not changed, and carmine was
taken with the meals to color the feces. Stool samples from

the last 4 days of the control period and the first 3 and
last 4 days of the bean-diet period were analyzed and the
data averaged. Of course, the limits of the different
periods were blurred in the stools and could be determined
only approximately (Table 9).

  Food intake differed widely among the test persons,
test subject B consuming the largest quantities, subject C
the smallest. The reactions of the various test subjects
to the beans meals, judged by the composition of their
stools, were quite individual. Although all the experimental subjects reacted to beans in their diet with a more
voluminous stool, caused by an increase in the daily output
of dry matter as well as of water (leading to the subjec-
tive comment that the urgency to motion was also increased),
the percentage of water in the stools did not vary accordingly. However, an increase of 2 to 3% in the water content represents a considerable softening and increase in
fluidity of the feces (62). Subjects B and C passed soft
stools already at the beginning of the experiment; consistency of the stools passed by subject C even markedly improved during the beans period.

  Persons B and D did not show the changes in feces production until the second bean-diet period. As the amount of
feces increased, so did the starch residue and fiber; the
starch residue was, however, only a very small portion of
bean starch consumed, about 70 g.

  The stools of test subjects A, B, and C showed a decreased pH, caused by an increase of lactic acid and the
volatile fatty acids; test subject D showed an increase only
in acetic acid. The increase in acid production while on
beans indicates that fermentation of carbohydrates had occurred in all test subjects. A slight increase in NH_3 production could be observed with persons C and D, indicating
some putrefaction of protein; accordingly, the drop in pH
of their feces on beans was only small.

  Moreover, our experiments show that basically, acid
production and gas production always take place, even after
intake of food low in fiber. The fear of fermentation in
the intestine--common among physicians--should thus be related only to excessive fermentation.

TABLE 9. Analytical Data Obtained from Feces Samples of Four Test Subjects while on a Control Diet and while on a Diet Including Beans (3d + 4d)

Test Subject	Period	Feces				pH	Lactic acid (mg/24h)	Volatile fatty acids $C_1/C_2/C_3/C_4$	Starch (g/24h)	Crude fiber (g/24h)	Protein (Nx6.25) (g/24h)	NH_3 (g/24h)
		Total g/24h	Dry Matter g/24h	Water g/24h	Water %							
A	Basal	157	37.7	1:9	75.8	7.0	61	23/343/112/127	0.8	4.3	21.25	114
	Beans (3d)	225	47.7	177	78.7	6.1	100	26/790/195/331	2.3	6.6	18.96	109
	Beans (4d)	106	27.1	79	74.5	6.7	35	11/386/95/144	0.5	2.8	11.41	62
B	Basal	397	64.5	332	83.6	6.7	69	8/510/205/274	2.9	14.2	22.81	88
	Beans (3d)	382	50.8	331	89.2	6.1	74	20/1007/382/341	1.5	9.6	19.37	75
	Beans (4d)	462	72.1	390	84.4	5.9	211	117/1524/467/543	3.0	14.1	21.06	81
C	Basal	81	13.1	68	84.0	7.3	20	10/200/59/59	0.3	1.2	5.94	23
	Beans (3d)	162	34.0	128	79.0	6.9	63	15/534/200/298	0.7	3.2	10.00	96
	Beans (4d)	128	31.6	96	75.0	7.1	58	11/439/126/129	0.5	2.5	10.64	82
D	Basal	90	22.2	68	75.5	7.2	78	23/629/180/215	0.9	2.7	10.31	60
	Beans (3d)	100	24.7	84	77.1	7.1	33	10/333/92/150	0.6	1.1	12.50	78
	Beans (4d)	135	33.1	102	75.6	6.8	51	37/2713/120/107	0.9	4.4	13.31	92

Source: Hellendoorn, 1969.

Note: Extreme values appearing in a bean-diet period are underlined.

Necessary investigations remaining to be done include determination of the IR of ingested food compared with that in the corresponding stools; in regard to various food products, what part will be found unfermented in the stool and what part is lost by fermentation.

Other observations confirm the view that bacteriological action is the primary cause for an increased intestinal transit rate after ingestion of high-residue food. This is demonstrated by the fact that guinea pigs reared free from microbes do not react on a fiber diet with increased peristalsis (37). People living on a synthetic diet of readily assimilable components show a reduced bacterial population in their bowel, scanty and infrequent bowel movements, and a sharp reduction in total fecal elimination (76); moreover, excessive fermentation gives rise to diarrhea (72).

A secondary question is: how do the fermentation acids stimulate the peristaltic movement of the gut responsible for accelerated transit? A direct pharmacodynamical stimulation on the intestinal wall has been suggested (70), but there is no proof of such an effect. However, investigations have made it appear more likely that the acids exert their influence by osmotic water binding (3, 4, 6).

The conception of water binding by fiber material itself, causing increased volume and water content of the stool, cannot hold, as the amount of fiber material is constantly diminishing from beginning to end of the digestive tract; the part of fiber that is left in the stool has the least water-binding capacity. On the other hand, fermentation acids are formed in the intestine, and their amount thus increases during bowel transit.

When the reduced intestinal transit time following the ingestion of high-residue food is discussed in the literature, it is not always clearly stated whether the transit referred to is through the small or the large intestine. However, the causes of accelerated transit through the small and large bowels are certainly different, although both types of transit originate from the ingestion of high-residue food.

As we have already shown, accelerated transit through the colon is a phenomenon that is principally bacteriologic in nature: unabsorbed carbohydrates serve as a substrate for fermentative reactions, the metabolites of which promote increased peristalsis. However, bacterial reactions are not involved in stimulating transit through the small bowel, except perhaps in the distal part. Here the fluid content of the food in the lumen during digestion is greatest, and bulking by water binding may exert its maximal effect. During passage through the colon, only those undigested components of fiber which resist bacterial breakdown may oppose desorption of water by their colloidal water-binding property (62). This effect, however, diminishes continuously during colon transit and is replaced by osmotic water binding by the low-molecular-weight products of bacterial metabolism.

Subjects on a diet containing whole-wheat bread show a small-bowel transit time 20% less than those on white bread (42). Moreover, stomach and small-bowel contents showed an increased bulk mainly caused by dilution of the food with saliva and gastric juice, the secretions of both being stimulated by more intensive chewing. However, it is questionable whether this effect of mastication on small-bowel transit, which is evident in the case of a semidry product such as bread, may be applied to all sorts of food products with a high-residue content. On the contrary, water content may be as important as fiber content. White bread, if toasted, must also be masticated thoroughly. In addition, beans and peas, for example, when cooked to softness, do not require much chewing before being swallowed. Neither is it necessary to chew intensively most vegetables that are cooked to a mushy consistency. The same applies to porridge of oat flakes. Thorough chewing remains necessary for most raw, firm fruits, raw vegetables, and nuts. Cooking increases their water content and destroys their cell structure, but may have only a minor effect on indigestible components.

As experimental data are still lacking, it remains uncertain whether vegetable foods, which have been cooked to softness and have attained maximal hydration, still exert a stimulating action on small-bowel transit. Closely related to the problem of the possibly accelerated transit of various high-residue foods through the small bowel is the question of possibly impaired absorption of nutrients and sterols.

VI. THE EFFECTS INTESTINAL BACTERIA AND FOOD RESIDUE EXERT ON EXCRETION OF STEROLS

Epidemiological studies show a lower prevalence of ischemic heart disease and generally lower serum lipid levels among people living in less industrialized communities than among those in Western societies. These differences have been attributed largely to dietary factors. Those people who have maintained their traditional food habits generally consume less saturated fat and less animal protein than is found in the Western diet. Moreover, their diet is based primarily on starchy foods with a high residue content. On the other hand, it has been assumed that the residue content of the diet of Westernized people having a high standard of living has decreased over the last century; this decrease has been attributed to changing food habits, mainly the present consumption of white bread and the high daily intake of sugar (6, 17). However, conclusions were based on crude-fiber values of the diets in question, as reliable figures on IR content of the diets are still lacking.

A possible influence of dietary fiber on cholesterol metabolism has attracted much attention during the last two decades (61). A hypocholesterolemic activity of several kinds of natural carbohydrate foods and some of their components has been demonstrated in experiments with animals, most of which had cholesterol-induced hypercholesterolemia. However, the results are not confined to cholesterol-fed animals (44). The results of experiments with human subjects are not always clear. For instance, the effect of whole-wheat bread or bran on blood lipids, as shown by the results of ten different investigations, is virtually nil (66). Rolled oats caused a small but significant reduction in serum cholesterol level (40). Leguminous seeds, when given over long periods of time and in quantities exceeding those of normal dietary habits, showed a marked hypocholesterolemic activity (25). Cellulose, an incomplete substitute for fiber, given in a high daily dose to children significantly lowered their blood cholesterol level (54). Of the food components, pectin clearly exhibits a serum-cholesterol-lowering activity (14, 29, 31, 50). When investigated, the reduction in serum cholesterol level was found to be attended by an increased excretion, mainly of acid sterols.

From the beginning, intestinal bacteria were surmised to play an important role in the disposal of steroids by way of the feces. Ahrens summarized the view as follows: "...it is apparent that the intestinal flora may affect serum cholesterol levels in at least two ways, (1) by converting cholesterol to a nonabsorbable compound, coprostanol, and (2) by degrading bile acids to products which are preferentially excreted in the feces, thus indirectly accelerating the conversion of cholesterol to bile acids" (1). Bulk was supposed to promote these bacterial reactions.

Our knowledge of cholesterol metabolism has meanwhile increased considerably (11, 16, 43). It is feasible to consider these bacterial reactions in greater detail. We shall see that the concept that bacteria has a direct influence on cholesterol metabolism cannot be maintained.

In regard to luminal cholesterol, we have to deal with cholesterol of both dietary and endogenous origin. The assumption is not quite true that, regardless of their quantitative importance, luminal sterols derived from the three major sources, diet, bile, and intestinal wall, would intermingle into a homogenous pool during the digestive process and would be absorbed to an equal extent.

Average dietary cholesterol intake in Western countries tends to be in the range of 150 to 350 mg/1000 cal (34), of which only a minor part is absorbed. Serum concentration in man is altered very little by cholesterol feeding, as absorption of dietary cholesterol remains limited to about 300 mg per day (11).

Small amounts of cholesterol synthesized in the liver are transported through the biliary tract and secreted into the duodenum. This endogenous cholesterol is efficiently taken up in segments of jejunum. However, cholesterol synthesis takes place not only in the liver, but to an appreciable extent also in the gastrointestinal tract itself, especially in the terminal ileum. Absorption of cholesterol, especially that of dietary and intestinal origin, is far from complete; its absorption is dependent on solubilization and the formation of mixed micelles by bile salts and such lipids as monoglyceride and fatty acid.

Nonabsorbed cholesterol is transported with the food residue to lower parts of the intestine and partly converted by bacteria into the two major fecal metabolites of cholesterol, coprostanol, and coprostanone. In general, unmetabolized cholesterol accounts for 25 to 45% of total fecal neutral steroid fraction; more than half of the neutral fecal sterols is in the form of coprostanol and a further 5 to 10% is usually in the form of coprostanone (12a).

The effect of differences in absorption of cholesterol from biliary and nonbiliary origin appears from the following studies.

As was shown by Danielsson, rats with ligated bile ducts excrete approximately the same amount of neutral sterols as do intact rats; considerable amounts of neutral sterols are also excreted in the feces of bile-fistula rats (10). Evidently, the neutral fecal sterols are to a considerable extent derived from nonbiliary sources. As cholesterol absorption takes place mainly in the upper part of the small intestine, reabsorption might primarily affect biliary cholesterol. Although many bacteria possess the ability to convert cholesterol, it is not likely that bacterial conversion of cholesterol, which takes place at more distal parts of the intestine, would be of great importance to cholesterol metabolism, since the bacteria are primarily converting dietary and intestinal cholesterol, which were to be lost in the feces anyway.

This view is supported by Kellogg and Wostmann (33). Although the excretion of neutral sterols by germ-free rats was found to be two thirds that of the conventional control rats, the opinion of those authors was that most of the increase in fecal neutral sterol excretion of the latter could be attributed to an increase in sloughing and/or secretion of sterols from the intestinal wall, rather than to the formation of unabsorbable neutral sterols by bacterial action.

Although cholesterol turnover in man is less influenced by excretion as bile acid (40%) than as neutral sterol (60%), yet excretion of bacterially degraded bile acids might be an important route for steroid disposal.

During enterohepatic circulation, synthesis from cholesterol of the primary bile salts, cholic acid and chenodeoxycholic acid, and conjugation of these acids with
taurine and glycine, takes place in the liver. The bile
salts are transported through the biliary tract and dis-
charged in the duodenum. After having assisted in lipid
digestion and absorption, the greater part is reabsorbed
in the lower ileum. The nonabsorbed bile salts are largely
deconjugated and dehydroxylated by intestinal bacteria,
predominantly into the secondary bile salts, deoxycholic
acid, and lithocholic acid, respectively. These reactions
take place in the terminal ileum and in the colon, where
bacteria are abundant. Deoxycholic acid, especially, is
largely absorbed in the colon, enters the portal vein, and
is transported to the liver. In the liver, reconjugation
occurs before joining recirculation together with the newly
synthesized conjugated primary bile salts. Lithocholic acid
and its conjugates, however, are highly insoluble, and only
minute amounts are absorbed; they are excreted almost completely with the feces, together with a great variety of
other degraded bile acids.

Only a small percentage, 5% at most, of luminal bile
salts escapes reabsorption during each enterohepatic recirculation. But, since the bile salt pool circulates six to
ten times each day, the cumulative daily loss from ileum to
colon is an appreciable proportion of the total bile salt
pool. The daily loss of bile acids in the feces of man is
approximately 200 to 600 mg (the total bile salt pool being
between 2.5 and 5.0 g). The size of the bile salt pool has
a pronounced effect on the rate of cholesterol absorption,
and it would alter, indirectly and primarily, the rate of
hepatic cholesterol synthesis.

In the gut, bacteria possessing the enzyme that is able
to deconjugate bile salts are widely distributed (12b).

More than 80% of the fecal bile acids have been 7
α-dehydroxylated (12b). Deoxycholic acid is the main constituent of fecal bile acids, and lithocholic acid can be
present in significant amounts (53).

Drasar and Hill, after having studied the production
of 7 α-dehydroxylase in vitro (12b), concluded that the
enzyme can be induced in 30 to 50% of strains of Bacteroides,

Bifidobacterium spp., and Clostridium spp., together with small numbers of Strep. fecalis and Veillonella spp. The conditions for production of the dehydroxylase, however, are rather stringent. It was found that the dehydroxylase is produced and active only under extremely anaerobic conditions. The enzyme is completely inducible by substrate; this might explain that the percentage of strict anaerobes able to 7 α-dehydroxylate increases with increasing fecal bile acid concentration. However, the enzyme is inhibited by substrate in excess of 6 mM (i.e., in excess of the normal level found in human feces).

Of particular interest for a possible influence of fermentation of undigested carbohydrates on cholesterol metabolism in man are the prerequisites that the dehydroxylase, which acts equally well on cholic as on chenodeoxycholic acid, have a pH optimum between 7 and 8, and that if the pH falls below 6.5 very little enzyme can be produced.

The higher degree of dehydroxylation of "English" compared with "Indian" and "Ugandan" fecal bile may thus be explained by differences in pH of the respective feces. Whereas the mean fecal pH of the English samples is 6.7 and 60% of them had a pH greater than 6.5, the mean fecal pH of the Ugandan samples was only 5.7 and less than 10% of them had a pH greater than 6.5 (12b).

Such a low pH of feces can be recorded only for people living on a high-residue diet that has a low animal protein content. The acids, formed in the large intestine by fermentation of undigested carbohydrates, tend to decrease the pH of feces. Alkaline degradation products of proteins tend to increase the pH of feces.

These facts might support the hypothesis that carcinogens are formed from deoxycholate in the etiology of colon cancer (27), but they are not compatible with the assumption that the increased steroid excretion following the intake of a diet with a high IR content might be caused by enhanced bacterial degradation of bile acids.

Experiments with germ-free and conventional animals on diets differing in residue content should provide us with a conclusive answer. Such a complete investigation with direct

determination of primary and degraded bile acids in feces
has not yet been carried out (15). Other investigations,
however, support the view that a secondary mechanism may
play a part in cholesterol metabolism.

Kellogg and Wostmann found the fecal excretion of bile
acids by conventional rats to be nearly twice as large as
that of germ-free rats; this ratio was in agreement with
the calculation that over 50% of bile acids excreted by
the conventional rats was bacterially modified, not including deconjugation (33). The authors did not identify the
factors responsible for the difference in bile acids excreted. However, it is possible that the bacterially modified bile acids were less readily absorbed than are the
primary and/or conjugated bile acids. This difference in
absorptive quality might be caused by the indirect influence
of bacteria on bile acid excretion, i.e., the binding of
the bacterially modified bile acids to bacteria, counter-
acting their absorption. In the colon it is probably a
major factor preventing reabsorption of degraded bile acids
(16a).

Binding of secondary bile acids by bacteria may account
for the higher percentage of the primary bile salts in bile
of baboons on a natural high-residue diet relative to those
on a semisynthetic diet. In addition, the baboons on the
natural diet showed a lower serum cholesterol content (36).
A similar shift in bile composition was found with volunteers eating bran and was observed in "Nigerian" bile vs
"English" bile (17).

A high-residue diet not only causes a shift in bile
salt composition of bile, but may have a pronounced influence on bile salt metabolism itself.

In animals, it has been shown that diets rich in refined
carbohydrates suppress the synthesis of bile salts in the
liver (17). Feeding bran to human subjects resulted in
marked reduction in circulating the deoxycholate pool, causing increased synthesis of chenodeoxycholate in the liver
and an increase in the pool of chenodeoxycholate. This proportion of the two bile salts suppresses the secretion of
cholesterol into bile (17, 51). Further studies showed that
"African" bile contains relatively more bile salts, less
deoxycholate, and less cholesterol than "British" bile (18).

Present knowledge makes it very likely that binding of the secondary bile acids in the colon has two important effects on hepatic cholesterol metabolism since (1) lithocholic acid has an inhibitory action on cholesterol catabolism (bile salt formation) in the liver, and (2) a high proportion of deoxycholic acid in respect to chenodeoxycholic acid stimulates cholesterol synthesis in the liver and hence its secretion into bile.

Thus, binding of the secondary bile acids in the colon ultimately results in a decreased cholesterol content of the liver. Obviously, metabolic processes governing lithogenic activity of bile largely coincide with those governing liver cholesterol content. In this context the latter may be of primary interest. However, a direct relationship between liver and plasma cholesterol content is not yet well established.

VII.   CONCLUSIONS

(1) Experiments with human subjects carried out in TNO's Central Institute for Nutrition and Food Research have demonstrated that some fermentation always occurs in the intestine, even on a low-residue Western diet. This fermentation results in organic acids in the stool, intestinal gas formation, and flatulence. By increasing the residue content of the diet (in our experiments the increase was obtained by substituting beans for white bread and potatoes), an increase in flatulence and in acid content of the stool could be observed; simultaneously, the volume and wet weight of the stool increased. In the experiments with animals, beans in the rations caused an increase in intestinal gas formation and accelerated transit of the food residue through the intestine.

(2) Fermentation in the lower intestine is attributed to bacterial degradation of the carbohydrates that have not been assimilated in the ileum, notably to the degradation of the fermentable carbohydrates of the indigestible residue of vegetable foods and possibly of some starch that has escaped digestion and absorption.

(3) The method for the determination of the indigestible residue of food is now available, so that, by analysis

of food ingested and of corresponding stools, the fermentable and nonfermentable parts of the indigestible residue
can be determined. The fermentable part of the indigestible food residue can provisionally be represented by the
difference between indigestible-residue content and crude-
fiber content of the food. Possibly the individual components of the indigestible food residue, and of the non-
fermented residue in the stool, may be determined by the
method given by Southgate. However, structural binding
properties are not elucidated by determination of the components.

(4) The variety in end products of fermentation results
from the character of the indigestible residue and from that
of the particular bacterial flora present in the various
segments of the gut of each individual subject. The end
products are the acids and gases in different relative
amounts. The character of the indigestible residue is determined by composition, incrustation, association, lignification, crystallinity, molecular weight, solubility, and fer-
mentability. Characteristics of the flora depend on the
dynamic ecosystem, formed by dietary and endogenous factors,
that governs the conditions for the various micro-organisms
to live in symbiosis. These two factors, indigestible residue and bacterial flora, ultimately determine the intestinal
segment in which final breakdown and formation of metabolic
end products takes place.

(5) The enhanced fecal steroid excretion after ingestion of a high-residue diet is probably not caused by
direct bacterial degradation of cholesterol or bile acids
and formation of nonabsorbable products. The increase of
steriods in the feces may be due to indirect action of bacteria, which may bind the secondary bile acids present in
the colon, thus indirectly influencing cholesterol metabolism. However, further investigation is necessary to prove
the validity of such a mechanism.

REFERENCES

1.   Ahrens, E. H., 1957, Nutritional factors and serum
     lipid levels, Am. J. Med., 23:928.

2. Am. Diet Assoc., 1971, Position paper on bland diet in
    the treatment of chronic duodenal ulcer disease (edi-
    torial), J. Am. Diet Assoc., 59:244.

3. Argenzio, R. A., Lowe, J. E., Pickard, D. W., and
    Stevens, C. E., 1974, Digesta passage and water ex-
    change in the equine large intestine, Am. J. Physiol.,
    226:1035.

4. Argenzio, R. A., Southworth, M., and Stevens, C. E.,
    1974, Sites of organic acid production and absorption
    in the equine gastrointestinal tract, Am. J. Physiol.,
    226:1043.

5. Berk, J. E. (ed.), 1968, Gastrointestinal gas, Ann.
    N. Y. Acad. Sci., 150:1.

6. Burkitt, D. P., Walker, A. R. P., and Painter, N. S.,
    1974, Dietary fiber and disease, J. Am. Med. Assoc.,
    229:1068.

7. Bustus Fernandez, L., Gonzales, E., Marzi, A., and
    Ledesma de Paolo, M. I., 1971, Fecal acidorrhea,
    New Engl. J. Med., 284:705.

8. Calloway, D. H., and Murphy, E. L., 1968, The use of
    expired air to measure intestinal gas production, Ann.
    N. Y. Acad. Sci., 150:82.

9. Christofaro, E., Mottu, F., and Wuhrmann, J. J.,
    "Involvement of the raffinose family of oligosaccharides
    in flatulence," in: Sugars in Nutrition, H. K. Sipple
    and K. W. McNutt, editors, (London: Academic Press, 1974)
    p. 313.

10. Danielson, H., 1960, On the origin of the neutral fecal
    sterols and their relation to cholesterol metabolism
    in the rat, Acta Physiol. Scand., 48:364.

11. Dietschy, J. M., and Wilson, J. D., 1970, Regulation
    of cholesterol metabolism, New Eng. J. Med., 282:1128,
    1179, 1241.

12. Drasar, B. S., and Hill, M. J., Human Intestinal Flora
    (London: Academic Press, 1974) (a) p. 124, (b) p. 103.

13. Eastwood, M. A., 1973, Vegetable fiber: its physical
     properties, Proc. Nutr. Soc., 32:137.

14. Grande, W., Anderson, J. F., and Keys, A., 1965, Effect
     of carbohydrates of leguminous seeds, wheat and pota-
     toes on serum cholesterol in man, J. Nutr., 86:313.

15. Gustafsson, B. E., and Norman, A., 1969, Influence of
     the diet on the turnover of bile-acids in germ-free and
     conventional rats, Br. J. Nutr., 23:429.

16. Heaton, K. W., Bile Salts in Health and Disease (Edin-
     burgh: Churchill Livingstone, 1972) p. 71.

17. Heaton, K. W., "Gallstones and Cholecystis," in: Refined
     Carbohydrate Foods and Disease, D. P. Burkitt and H. C.
     Trowell, editors, (London: Academic Press, 1975) p. 173.

18. Heaton, K. W., Wicks, A. C. B., and Yeats, J., Bile
     composition in relation to race and diet: Studies in
     Rhodesian Africans and in British subjects, Interna-
     tional Bile Acid Meeting, Basle, October 1976.

19. Hellendoorn, E. W., 1969, Intestinal effects following
     ingestion of beans, Food Techn., 23:87.

20. Hellendoorn, E. W., 1971, Aspects of retrogradation in
     some dehydrated starch containing precooked food pro-
     ducts, Stärke, 23:63.

21. Hellendoorn, E. W., "Enzymatic determination of insolu-
     ble, indigestible residue of beans," in: Nutritional
     Improvement of Food Legumes by Breeding, M. Milner,
     editor, Proceedings of a Symposium, Rome, July 1972.
     New York, PAG, 1973, p. 321.

22. Hellendoorn, E. W., 1973, Physiological importance of
     indigestible carbohydrates in human nutrition, Voeding,
     34:618.

23. Hellendoorn, E. W., "Carbohydrate digestibility and
     flatulence activity of beans," in: Nutritional Aspect
     of Common Beans and Other Legume Seeds as Animal and
     Human Food, W. G. Jaffé, editor, proceedings of a meet-
     ing, Ribeirao Preto, Brazil, November 1973. Caracas:
     Sociedad Latinoamericanos de Nutricion, 1975, p. 261.

24. Hellendoorn, E. W., 1975, Enzymatic determination of
     the indigestible residue (dietary fibre) content of
     human food, J. Sci. Food Agric., 26:1461.

25. Hellendoorn, E. W., 1976, Beneficial physiological
     action of beans, J. Am. Diet. Assoc., 69:248.

26. Hellendoorn, E. W., van den Top, M., and van der Weide,
     J. E. M., 1970, Digestibility in vitro of dry mashed
     potato products, J. Sci. Food Agric., 21:71.

27. Hill, M. J., 1974, Steroid nuclear dehydrogenation and
     colon cancer, Am. J. Clin. Nutr., 27:1475.

28. Horwitz, W., editor, Official methods of analysis
     of the Association of Official Analytical Chemists,
     11th ed., Washington, D.C., 1970.

29. Informatics. Scientific literature reviews on generally
     recognized as safe (Gras) food ingredients. Pectin.
     Prepared for Food and Drug Administration; distributed
     by NTIS: PB-230306, Rockville, Maryland, 1974.

30. Jackel, S. S., Schultz, A. S., and Schraeder, W. E.,
     1953, Susceptibility of the starch in fresh and stale
     bread to enzymatic digestion, Science, 118:18.

31. Jenkins, D. J. A., Leeds, A. R., Newton, C., and Cum-
     mings, J. H., 1975, Effect of pectin, guar-gum, and
     wheat fibre on serum-cholesterol, Lancet, 1:1116.

32. Katz, J. R., 1934, Über den Zusammenhang der Änderungen
     der Stärke beim Altbacken werden des Brotes und beim
     Retrogradieren von Stärkekleister, Z. Physik. Chemie A.,
     169:321.

33. Kellogg, T. F., and Wostmann, B. S., 1969, Fecal neutral
     steroids and bile acids from germfree rats, J. Lipid Res.,
     10:495.

34. Keys, A., Anderson, J. T., and Grande, F., 1965, Serum
     cholesterol response to changes in the diet, II. The
     effect of cholesterol in the diet, Metabolism, 14:759.

35. Kim, W. J., Smit, C. J. B., and Nakayama, T. O. M.,
     1973, The removal of oligosaccharides from soybeans,
     Lebensm.-Wiss. Technol., 6:201.

36. Kritchevsky, D., Tepper, S. A., and Story, J. A.,
     1975, Non-nutritive fiber and lipid metabolism,
     J. Food Sci., 40:8.

37. Kuhn, R., 1954, Probleme des keimfreien Lebens,
     Naturwiss. Rundsch., 7:445.

38. Levitt, M. D., 1972, Intestinal gas production, J. Am.
     Diet Assoc., 60:487.

39. Lüder, W., Aust, L., and Vetter, K., 1969, Zum Verlauf
     der alimentären Hyperglykämie nach Brotverzehr, Nahrung,
     13:191.

40. Luyken, R., de Wijn, J. F., Pikaar, N. A., and van der
     Meer, R., 1965, De invloed van havermout op het serum-
     cholesterolgehalte van het bloed, Voeding, 26:229.

41. McCance, R. A., Prior, K. M., and Widdowson, E. M.,
     1953, A radiological study of the rate of passage of
     brown and white bread through the digestive tract of
     man, Br. J. Nutr., 7:98.

42. McCance, R. A., and Widdowson, E. M., 1960, The compo-
     sition of foods, 3rd Ed. Spec. Rept. Sr. No. 297,
     London, Medical Research Council.

43. McIntyre, H., and Isselbacher, K. J., 1973, Role of the
     small intestine in cholesterol metabolism, Am. J. Clin.
     Nutr., 26:647.

44. Mokady, S., 1973, Effect of dietary pectin and algin on
     blood cholesterol level in growing rats fed a choles-
     terol-free diet, Nutr. Metab., 15:250.

45. Murphy, E. L., 1964, Flatus. Conference on nutrition
     in space and related waste problems, Tampa: University
     of South Florida, p. 255.

46. Murphy, E. L., 1964, The isolation and testing of the
     flatulence factor in gas-forming foods. Proceedings
     of the Seventh Annual Research Conference on Dry Beans
     (Ithaca and Geneva), ARS 74-32:45.

47. Murphy, E. L., 1969, What do we know about flatulence
     in 1968? Proceedings of the Ninth Annual Research
     Conference on Dry Beans (Fort Collins), ARS 74-50:86.

48. Murphy, E. L., Horsley, H., and Burr, H. K., 1972,
     Fractionation of dry bean extracts which increase
     carbon dioxide egestion in human flatus, J. Agric.
     Food Chem., 20:813.

49. Norman, A. G., The Biochemistry of Cellulose, the Poly-
     uronides, Lignin, Etc., (Oxford: Clarendon Press, 1937)
     p. 39.

50. Palmer, G. H., and Dixon, D. G., 1966, Effect of pectin
     dose on serum cholesterol levels, Am. J. Clin. Nutr.,
     18:437.

51. Pomare, E. W., Heaton, K. W., Low-Beer, T. S., and
     Espiner, H. J., 1976, The effect of wheat bran upon
     bile salt metabolism and upon the lipid composition of
     bile in gallstone patients, Digest. Dis., 21:521.

52. Rogols, S., and Meites, S., 1968, The effect of starch
     species on alpha-amylase activity, Stärke, 20:256.

53. Rosenfeld, R. S., and Hellmann, L., 1962, Excretion of
     steroid acids in man, Arch. Biochem. Biophys., 97:406.

54. Shurpalekar, K. S., Doraiswamy, T. R., Sundaravalli,
     O. E., and Narayana Rao, M., 1971, Effect of inclusion
     of cellulose in an "atherogenic" diet on the blood
     lipids of children, Nature, 232:554.

55. Southgate, D. A. T., 1969, Determination of carbohydrates
     in foods, II. Unavailable carbohydrates, J. Sci. Food
     Agric., 20:331.

56. Southgate, D. A. T., and Durnin, J. V. G. A., 1970,
     Caloric conversion factors. An experimental reassess-
     ment of the factors used in the calculation of the
     energy value of human diets, Br. J. Nutr., 24:517.

57. Spiller, G. A., and Amen, R. J., 1975, Plant fibers in
     nutrition: need for better nomenclature. Letter to
     the editor, Am. J. Clin. Nutr., 28 (7):674.

58. Stanway, A., Taking the Rough with the Smooth (London:
     Souvenir Press, 1976).

59. Steggerda, F. R., 1963, Effect of certain drugs on
     flatus production while on beans. Proceedings of the
     Sixth Annual Conference on Dry Beans (Los Angeles),
     p. 28.

60. Steggerda, F. R., 1964, The mechanism of gas production
     following the consumption of beans. Proceedings of
     the Seventh Annual Research Conference on Dry Beans
     (Ithaca and Geneva), ARS 74-32:56.

61. Story, J. A., and Kritchevsky, D., "Dietary fiber and
     lipid metabolism," in: Fiber in Human Nutrition, G. A.
     Spiller and R. J. Amen, editors, (New York: Plenum,
     1976), chapter 7.

62. Tainter, M. L., and Buchanan, O. H., 1954, Quantitative
     comparison of colloidal laxatives, Ann. N. Y. Acad.
     Sci., 58:438.

63. Thomas, B., and Winkler, S., 1968, Zur Problem der
     quantitativen Stärkeanalytik, Stärke, 20:332.

64. Tropp, C., 1950, Untersuchungen über die Bekömmlichkeit
     des Brotes, Getreide, Mehl, Brot, 4:267.

65. Trowell, H., 1974, Definitions of fibre, Lancet, 1:503.

66. Truswell, A. S., and Kay, R. M., 1976, Bran and blood-
     lipids, Lancet, 1:367.

67. Van de Kamer, J. H., and van Ginkel, L., 1952, Rapid
     determination of crude fibre (cellulose) in cereals,
     Cereal Chem., 29:239.

68. Van Deventer, W. H., and Pilnik, W., 1976, Fractiona-
     tion of pectins in relation to their degree of esteri-
     fication, Lebensm.-Wiss. Technol., 9:42.

69. Van Soest, P. J., and McQueen, R. W., 1973, The chemistry and estimation of fiber, Proc. Nutr. Soc., 32:123.

70. Weinstein, L., et al., 1961, Diet as related to gastrointestinal function, J. Am. Med. Assoc., 176:935.

71. Weijers, H. A., and van de Kamer, J. H., 1965, Alteration of intestinal bacterial flora as a cause of
diarrhoea, Nutr. Abstr. Rev., 45:591.

72. Weyers, H. A., van de Kamer, J. H., Wauters, E. A. K.,
and Pikaar, N. A., 1971, Diagnosis of malabsorption.
Proceedings of XIII International Congress of Pediatrics,
Vienna, p. 13.

73. Williams, R. D., and Olmsted, W. H., 1935, A biochemical
method for determining indigestible residue (crude fiber)
in feces: lignin, cellulose, and non-watersoluble hemicellulose, J. Biol. Chem., 108:653.

74. Williams, R. D., and Olmsted, W. H., 1936, Effect of
cellulose, hemicellulose and lignin on weight of stool.
A contribution to the study of laxation in man, J. Nutr.,
11:433.

75. Williams, R. D., and Olmsted, W. H., 1936, The manner
in which food controls the bulk of the feces, Ann.
Intern. Med., 10:718.

76. Winitz, M., et al., 1970, Studies in metabolic nutrition employing chemically defined diets, Amer. J. Clin.
Nutr., 23:525.

CHAPTER 7

PRACTICAL DIETARY RESEARCH DESIGN AND APPLICATIONS

FOR SOUTHWESTERN AMERICAN INDIANS

Margaret E. Hendrikx

National Institute of Arthritis,
Metabolism, and Digestive Diseases

Phoenix, Arizona

I. INTRODUCTION

Some of the practical problems in planning human research studies on effects of fiber feeding are the selection
of type and amount of fiber, dietary calculation of the
fiber and nutrients, patient acceptance, study duration,
and differences in populations. In both planning and evaluation of research, there are difficulties in interpretation
of the literature because of differences in terminology and
analytic technique.

II. FIBER SELECTION

The fiber chosen will depend on the attributes needed
for the study and on the acceptibility of flavor, texture,
form, and dose size. Some characteristics of fiber which
have been studied include (1) binding capacity for bile acids,
ammonia, and carcinogens and (2) effects on serum cholesterol and triglycerides. The dietary composition may alter
the extent of binding by fiber. Whyte observed a decreased
reabsorption of bile acids on low-fat, high-carbohydrate
diets (38). Complex carbohydrate diets, low in fat and cholesterol, decreased serum triglycerides but not serum cholesterol. The ratio of polyunsaturated to saturated fat
may also alter test results of diets containing a significant
amount of fat.

Characteristics of the various fibers must be assessed. Lignin, which has been called a bile-salt-sequestering agent, is resistant to microbial action in vitro (11). Unfortunately, diets containing a significant proportion of lignin may produce constipation and a slow transit time, allowing greater digestion of cellulose and hemicellulose (10). Vegetable fibers have proven useful in some studies, but when maximal bulk in the colon and intestine is required, a slowly digested fiber is indicated. Digestion of the cell wall material of many common vegetables is extraordinarily rapid, with 90% of maximum digestion occurring before 15 hr (35). Lesser digestibility of the cell wall is related to high lignin: cellulose ratios. In this respect, bran has a higher ratio than legumes, cauliflower, rutabaga, potatoes, carrots, apples, lettuce, onions, and oranges. The fiber of less mature fruits and vegetables is digested even more rapidly than the fiber of those fully developed. This variability and the rapid digestion time render vegetable fibers less effective than bran for maximal colon bulk. Decreased particle size enhances digestibility, but for bran, this is probably more than offset by the increased rate of passage caused by residual fiber.

The dose size can be planned to be sufficient to elicit change, if one is possible, and then titrated to the minimal quantity that results in the desired change. Although no severe adverse effects of a high-fiber diet have been reported, there have been cases of temporary paradoxical constipation. Crane et al. reported that two patients receiving short-chained methylcellulose had fluid retention, which was reversed when the cellulose feeding was withdrawn (5). Increased stool volume is to be expected and diarrhea may occur with fiber feeding. The discomfort of abdominal distention can be alleviated by daily ingestion of small amounts of fiber and gradual increases until the desired level of intake is reached. Maximal human tolerance for fiber is unknown, but in our preliminary studies most healthy volunteers consumed over 100 g of bran daily for 1 month. The limitation thus far has not been due to tolerance level, but to the need to maintain constant weight on balance studies. The caloric total of an adequate base diet incorporating 100 g of bran has been adequate to maintain weight for some patients.

A concentrated source of fiber is advantageous when
large quantities are required or when the fiber must be
mixed with other foods. Food fibers have been recommended
as preferable to wood cellulose or synthetic fibers (5,23).
For example, bran has been shown to improve glucose tolerance
while wood cellulose does not (21). Similarly, rats fed
alfalfa or cellulose showed lowered serum and liver cholesterol levels only with alfalfa (22). In-vitro experiments
with dry grain, a maize and barley byproduct of whisky malt-
ings, showed a considerable affinity of lignin for bile salts
and acids at acid pH (12). For long-term restricted feeding programs, legumes and other vegetables are bulky, monot-
onous, and difficult to incorporate in many forms. Unprocessed or baker's bran has been widely used and has some
advantages. Generally low in cost, it is widely available
and mixes well with other foods in raw or cooked form. These
qualities also enhance its use for therapeutic regimes.

III. DIETARY CALCULATION

Estimation of the nutrient intake from ingested bran
is problematic, as is the calculation of the expected amount
of indigestible fiber. Standard reference tables show 59
to 60% availability of total caloric value but do not indicate individual nutrient availability (24,37). Laboratory
analysis of both crude protein and fiber-bound protein is
necessary for the estimation of the protein potentially
available. Although fat comprises only 3 to 5% of bran on
analysis, its higher caloric value can lead to overestimation
of energy intake if the bound complex lipid fraction is unknown. Since 12 hr are required for completion of 98% of
the digestion and absorption of fat in the small intestine,
variation in individual transit times may also alter availability. Fiber may limit the rate of energy absorption and
the conversion of carbohydrate to fat (20). The decrease in
dietary digestibility is restricted to lessened absorption
of the fat, nitrogen, and energy of the fiber itself.

Regardless of whether limitations of digestion of the
cell-wall carbohydrates are caused by shortened transit time
or by lignin, tannins, or other substances with anticellulase
activity, the hemicellulose and cellulose appear to be more
fully digested than most standard nutrition texts indicate
(9,14,16). Carbohydrate, in the form of hemicellulose and

cellulose, comprises a significant proportion (56%) of bran
and, therefore, a substantial part of the intake on high-
bran diets (29). One indication of nutrient availability
is weight maintenance during balance studies, with and without bran. A diet calculated on assumed nutritional value
of bran can be substituted isocalorically for a lower fiber
balance diet and weight maintained. A presumed absorption
rate can be used to estimate available carbohydrate. The
human absorption figures of Crampton and Maynard (4), 38%
for cellulose and 56% for hemicellulose (Table 1), are some-
what different from the rates for dogs of 50 to 70% for
cellulose and 20 to 50% for hemicellulose (36). Absorption
of lignin is questionable but probably negligible during
the transit times of 48 hr or less, which would be expected
on a high-fiber diet.

This sample would then be calculated as yielding 68.6
calories as carbohydrate from the cellulose and hemicellulose
and containing 18.34 g of unavailable fiber per 100 g. This
is higher than the 8.24 g of crude fiber analyzed from the
same product, but lower than the estimation from in-vitro
digestion by rumen bacteria. This showed approximately 56%
undigested in 24 hr and 51% at 48 hr (28). The calculated
available carbohydrate fraction, together with the corrected
protein and fat figures, can be used to plan isocaloric substitution of bran for weight maintenance. The hemicellulose,
cellulose, and lignin figures can be reported individually
as suggested by Spiller and Amen (32).

IV.   DIETARY DESIGN

Hemicellulose, cellulose, and lignin are neither bio-
logically nor chemically similar in different plant materials (35). To test the effect of a fiber source, the other
constituents of the diet must be low in fiber. This increases the monotony of the usual rigid, repetitive long-term
diet required for many research studies. Careful patient
selection and explanation of the purpose and restrictions
of the diet can promote adherence to the regime.

If only small amounts of fiber are to be fed daily,
it may be given at a single meal; but if large amounts are
to be ingested, divided doses throughout the day aid in
avoiding abdominal distention. Some investigators utilize

Table 1. Sample Calculation of Carbohydrate Availability
From the Cellulose and Hemicellulose of Bran

Bran	Hemi cellu- lose	Cellu- lose	Lignin	Total
g/100 g, analyzed moisture corrected	25.81	7.13	2.56	35.50
Percent available	56.00	38.00	--	--
g/100 g available	14.45	2.71	--	17.16
Percent unavailable	44.00	62.00	--	--
g/100 g unavailable	11.36	4.42	2.56	18.34
g available ± g unavailable	--	--	--	35.50

Source: Crampton and Maynard (3).

only raw bran (18), but greater variety can be offered by
using both raw and cooked foods incorporating bran. One or
two tablespoons (3 to 8 g) of bran are easily added to standard servings of dry or cooked cereals and soups. Similar
amounts can be given in pancakes, biscuits, quick breads,
or muffins. Eight g of bran can be contained in 90 g of
ground beef, with the addition of water if the mixture is
dry. Since it lacks gluten, bran requires a binding agent
when used as a coating in place of flour or as a substitute
for bread crumbs. Most standard bread recipes can be adapted to incorporate bran in addition to or as part of the flour.
A lighter, higher loaf is usually obtained if bran is added
after the dough has once risen and gluten strands developed.
When bran is used as a sweet as cookies, macaroons, or pud-
ding, its natural flavor is enhanced by addition of almond
or other nut flavorings. A four-meal plan incorporating
25 to 50 g of bran per meal has been acceptable to our
patients. This is enhanced by presenting the bran in a variety of ways.

V. DIFFERENCES IN POPULATIONS

World-wide differences among populations in disease incidence and fiber intake have been linked epidemiologically (25). Clinical research in metabolic differences of populations is less well explored. Groups with conditions that may be influenced by fiber ingestion provide a more meaningful study area than subjects with normal biological values that are unlikely to be influenced (19,34). Some studies on the effects of fiber feeding have been conducted in Caucasian groups at high risk for serum cholesterol and triglyceride elevations, diverticular disease, and colon cancer. Not all populations exhibit these characteristics and, for these groups, evaluation of the effects of fiber on serum glucose and bile acids may be of greater importance.

One such population includes some of the southwestern American Indian tribes. Compared to United States standards, they have been characterized as having low serum cholesterol levels; an increased prevalence of diabetes mellitus, gall-stones, and obesity; and decreased frequency of duodenal ulcer, colon cancer, and atherosclerosis (30). In controlled studies of Indian women with cholesterol gallstones, the biliary output of bile acids was decreased and secretion of biliary cholesterol increased (15). The increase in biliary cholesterol may be partially due to obesity of the subjects, but the condition presents an interesting model for fiber feeding. As reported by Pomare and Heaton and confirmed by Falaiye, bran or fiber feeding reduces the degradation of bile salts by colonic bacteria (13,26).

The first study used 33+10 g bran per day and produced halving of the deoxycholate portion of the bile salt pool from 27.1+8.9% to 13.8+4.2%. This reduction was matched by an increase in the proportion of chenodeoxycholate from 30.6+3.6% to 43.9+2.7%. The proportion of cholate remained unchanged at 42.2%. A suggested mechanism is inhibition of 7-alpha dehydroxylation by bran (27). Ingestion of approximately 500 mg of chenodeoxycholate daily increased the proportion of chenodeoxycholate in the bile from 34.8+1.4% to 73.1+3.1%, while deoxycholic acid decreased from 23.8+2.6% to 4.9+1.4% (1). The decrease in lithogenicity of the bile which accompanies chenodeoxycholate feeding was primarily due to decreased biliary cholesterol secretion, with no decrease in fecal excretion. This suggests a method for dissolution of cholesterol gallstones (8). If fiber feeding

could produce similar results without the possible side
effects of bile salt feeding--diarrhea, hypercholesterolemia,
and hepatotoxicity (3)--it might be of value for populations
with a high incidence of cholesterol gallstone formation.

Population differences in fecal excretion may be significant. In studies using a diet containing 40% fat, normal male Indians excreted more steroids than Caucasians (28).
Comparing daily output in mg per 70 kg of body weight,
Indians excreted 425 mg of acidic steroids and Caucasians
247 mg; for neutral steroids, Indians 1057 mg and Caucasians
679 mg. Total steroid excretion was 1483 mg for Indians
and 941 mg for Caucasians. Although increased fecal steroids
have been linked to carcinoma of the colon in some groups (7),
this condition is rare in southwestern Indians. In this study
there were significant differences in stool weight. For
comparison, fullblooded Pima, Papago, and Hopi Indians and
Caucasians were fed a low-residue diet containing 15% protein and 40% fat (lard as the principle source), with
caloric adjustment to maintain weight. As shown in Table 2,
all groups on the low-residue diet had below-average standard
stool weight. Both male and female Caucasians were within
normal ranges, but neither Indian group attained the lowest
standard range figure. This was most marked in the Indian
males, which was the group with the heaviest body weight.
Corrected to an average of 70 kg body weight, the Indian
males had the lowest average stool weight of the four groups.
This was even lower than a 65.3 g average fecal mass for
patients on elemental diets (6).

Overlapping of body, stool, and range of stool weights
was more frequent for females than males. Average stool
weight for the 22 Caucasians was 95.28 g and for the 17
Indians 76.5 g, a difference of 18.78 g.

VI. CONCLUSION

Significant differences occur between races and sex
and race, though not sex alone. In tribal groups excreting
smaller stools than Caucasians on the same diet, studies on
the effect of fiber may prove of interest.

There have been reports that fiber feeding may reduce
serum glucose levels (21), the incidence of diabetes (33),

TABLE 2. Comparison of Average Stool Weight per 24 Hours for Indians and Caucasians

Race	Male				Female			
	Number Patients	Number Stools	Stool Weight (g)		Number Patients	Number Stools	Stool Weight (g)	
			Range	Av/70 kg Body Wt			Range	Av/70 kg Body Wt
Indian	8	210	3-348	63.52	9.	132	7-205	73.23
Caucasian	5	174	7-438	110.28	17	385	1-398	90.35

Comparison of Stool Wt in Grams to Standard[1]

Race	Male				Female			
	Av Body Wt (kg)	Av Wt Stool (g)	Standard Stool Wt for Given Body Wt		Av Body Wt (kg)	Av Wt Stool (g)	Standard Stool Wt for Given Body Wt	
			Average	Range			Average	Range
Indian	84.70	76.86	148.99	88.94-201.59	72.83	76.19	128.11	.76.47-173.34
Caucasian	76.52	120.55	134.60	80.35-182.12	68.06	87.85	119.82	71.46-161.98

[1]Altman and Dittmer (2).

and the extent of obesity (17). These might also prove of
interest for study among southwestern American Indians in
whom more than half of those over age 15 years exceed ideal
weight by greater than 25% (31). For the tribes with high
rates of obesity and diabetes such as exists among the Pima,
Papago, and Colorado River tribes, such studies may have
even greater relevance (30).

If prospective research can be designed to compare the
type and amount of fiber ingested with the subsequent disease
or physical status, it may aid in clarification of the roles
of fiber in human nutrition.

REFERENCES

1.   Adler, R. D., Bennion, L. J., Duane, W. C. and
      Grundy, S. M., 1975, Effects of low-dose chenodeoxy-
      cholic acid feeding on biliary lipid metabolism,
      Gastroenterology, 68:326.

2.   Altman, P. L., Dittmer, D. S., 1968, Metabolism, Fed.
      Am. Soc. Exptl. Biol., Besthesda, Md., p. 515.

3.   Bell, G. D., 1974, The present position concerning
      gallstones dissolution, Gut., 15:913.

4.   Crampton, E. W. and Maynard, L. A., 1938, The relation
      of cellulose and lignin content to the nutritive value
      of animal feeds, J. Nutr., 15:383.

5.   Crane, Milton, G., Harris, J. J., Herber, R., Shankel, S.
      and Specht, N., 1969, Excessive fluid retention related
      to cellulose ingestion: studies on two patients,
      Metabolism, 18:945.

6.   Crowther, J. S., Drasar, B. S., Goddard, P., Hill, M. J.
      and Johnson, K., 1973, The effect of a chemically
      defined diet on faecal flora and faecal steroid con-
      centration, Gut., 14:790.

7.   Cummings, J. H., 1973, Progress report on dietary
      fiber, Gut., 14:69.

8.   Danzinger, R. G., Hofmann, A. F., Schoenfield, L. J.,
     and Thistle, J. L., 1972, Dissolution of cholesterol
     gallstones by chenodeoxycholic acid, N. Eng. J. Med.,
     286:1.

9.   Davidson, S., and Passmore, R., Human Nutrition and
     Dietetics, 4th edition (Philadelphia: Lea and Febiger,
     1973).

10. Eastwood, M. A., and Girwood, R. H., 1964, The mean-
     ing of high- and low-residue diets, Gastroenterology,
     47:649.

11. Eastwood, M. A., and Girwood, R. H., 1968, Lignin:
     a bile-salt sequestering agent, Lancet, 2:1170.

12. Eastwood, M. A., and Hamilton, D., 1973, Studies on
     the absorption of bile salts to nonabsorbed components
     of the diet, Biochimica et Biophysica Acta, 152:165.

13. Falaiye, J. M., 1974, Bile salt patterns in Nigerians
     on a high-fibre diet, Lancet, 1:1002.

14. Goodhart, R. S., and Shils, M. D., Modern Nutri-
     tion in Health and Disease, 5th edition, (Philadelphia:
     Lea and Febiger, 1973) p. 102.

15. Grundy, S. M., Metzger, A. L., and Adler, R. D., 1972,
     Mechanisms of lithogenic bile formation in American
     Indian women with and without cholesterol gallstones,
     J. of Clin. Invest., 51:3026.

16. Guthrie, H. A., Introductory Nutrition (St. Louis:
     C. V. Mosby, 1971) p. 25.

17. Heaton, K. W., 1973, Food fibre as an obstacle to energy
     intake, Lancet, 2:1418.

18. Heaton, K. W., and Pomare, E. W., 1974, Effect of bran
     on blood lipids and calcium, Lancet, 1:49.

19. Heaton, K. W., and Pomare, E. W., 1975, Bran and blood
     lipids, Lancet, 5:800.

20. James, W. P. T., and Cummings, J. H., 1974, Dietary fibre and energy regulation, Lancet, 1:61.

21. Jeffrys, D. B., 1974, The effect of dietary fibre on the response to orally administered glucose, Proc. of the Nutr. Soc., 33:11A.

22. Kritchevsky, D., 1974, Isocaloric, isogravic diets in rats, III, Nutr. Rep. Int., 9:301.

23. Kritchevsky, D., and Story, J. A., 1974, Binding of bile salts in vitro by nonnutritive fiber, J. Nutr., 104:458.

24. Leung, W. W., Butrum, R. R., and Chang, F. H., 1972, Food composition table for use in East Asia, Pub. No. 73, (NIH), p. 9, DHEW.

25. Medical World News, Roughage in the diet, September 6, 1974, 35.

26. Pomare, E. W., and Heaton, K. W., 1973, Alteration of bile salt metabolism by dietary fibre (bran), Brit. Med. J., 4:262.

27. Reilly, R., and Kirsner, J. B., 1975, Fiber deficiency and colonic disorders, Am. J. Clin. Nutr., 28:293.

28. Robertson, J. B., 1975, Personal communication.

29. Saunders, R. M. and Walker, H. G., 1969, The sugars of wheat bran, Cereal Chemistry, 46:85.

30. Sievers, M. L., 1966, Disease patterns among southwestern Indians, P. H. Reports, 81:1075.

31. Sievers, M. L., and Hendrikx, M. E., 1972, Two weight-reduction programs among southwestern Indians, Health Services Reports, 87:530.

32. Spiller, G. A., and Amen, R. J., 1974, Research on dietary fibre, Lancet, 2:1259.

33. Trowell, H., 1974, Diabetes mellitus death rates in England and Wales, 1920-1970, and food supplies, Lancet, 2:998.

34.   Trowell, H., 1975, Bran and blood lipids, Lancet, $\underline{5}$:801.

35.   Van Soest, P. J., and McQueen, R. W., 1973, Symposium
      on fibre in human nutrition, Proceedings of the Nutri-
      tion Society, $\underline{32}$:123.

36.   Visek, W. J., and Robertson, J. B., 1973, Cornell
      Nutrition Conference, p. 18.

37.   Watt, B. K., and Merrill, A. L., 1963, Composition of
      foods, raw, processed and prepared, Ag. Handbook No. 8,
      p. 66.

38.   Whyte, H. M., Nestel, P. J., and Pryke, E. S., 1973,
      Bile acid and cholesterol excretion with carbohydrate-
      rich diets, J. Lab. Clin. Med., $\underline{81}$:818.

CHAPTER 8

PALEODIETETICS: A REVIEW OF THE ROLE OF DIETARY FIBER

IN PREAGRICULTURAL HUMAN DIETS

Michael Kliks

Division of Entomology and Parasitology
University of California

Berkeley, California

I.   INTRODUCTION

In a biochemical and physiological sense man is not a
particularly "modern" animal. Rather, he shares many
adaptive mechanisms which were already established several
million years ago during the lower Pleistocene era in early
homonids, most of which were predominantly herbivorous (26,
46, 52, 57), as is the case today. The manifold physiochemi-
cal functions of dietary fiber in human digestive and excretory processes certainly did not develop de novo in man, but
were common to all higher primates and many other monogastric
terrestrial vertebrates as well (6, 34). These processes and
the basic architecture of the gastrointestinal tract quite
probably evolved over several hundred thousand generations
in response to the continuous, selective pressures of a
broadly based but consistently phytic diet (17, 19, 39). It
is now apparent that during the last 20,000 years, the human
diet has undergone a series of far reaching "revolutions,"
the overall trend of which has been away from a coarse,
plant-based regime of foraged leafy greens, seeds, stalks,
roots, flowers, and other tissues, to a more limited, often
monotypic, diet based primarily on a few cereal grains,
tubers, and legumes (Figure 1). The importance of the former diet, that of the hunter-gatherer, in shaping the structure and function of the human gastrointestinal tract can
hardly be overestimated.

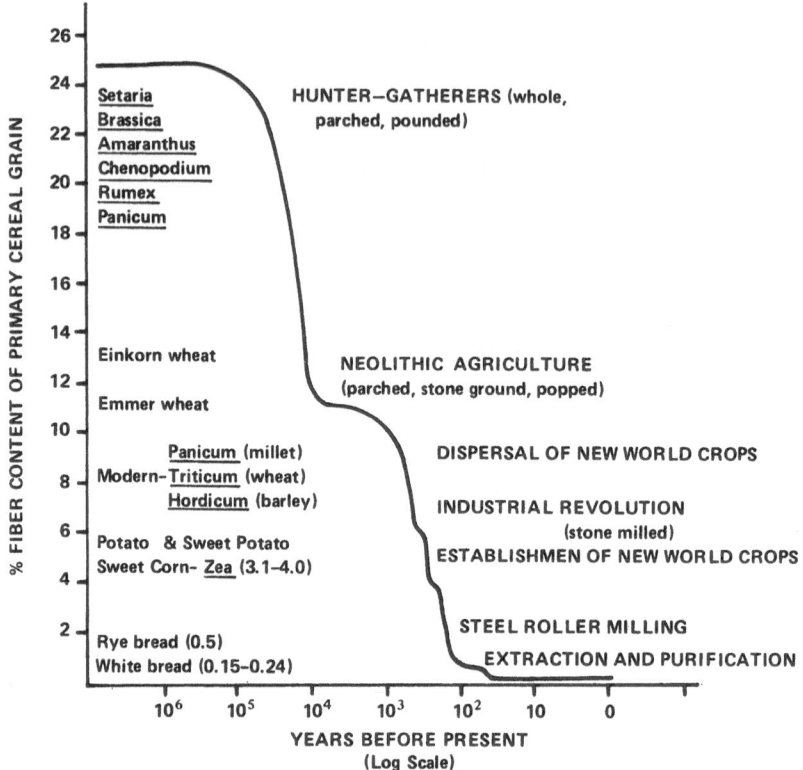

Figure 1. Change in fiber content of Old World primary cereal grains.

Advances in the elucidation of the nature and range of early human dietary regimes should be of great interest, therefore, to those who wish to understand the ontogony and pathogenesis of the many diseases of contemporary man that have been linked to deficiencies in dietary fiber intake (5, 6, 18). The importance of studies of pongid primate diet (66) and gastrointestinal tract structure, function (4, 61), and pathobiology, both in nature and in the laboratory, should be widely recognized, although few references to such work exist in the current literature.

Until recently, all speculation as to the nature of the early human diet has been based on the indirect evidence

of food remains recovered in archaeological contexts (33, 51)
or on cursory, uncontrolled observations of the dietary intakes of existing primitive human groups of hunter-gatherers
(43, 47, 54, 64, 67, 79) and incipient agriculturalists (1,
2, 19, 50, 53, 78). Both of these sources of information
suffer from serious deficiencies that greatly restrict their
usefulness in proposing meaningful reconstructions of the
total dietary constituents of early or primitive man.

Prior to the recognition of the importance of analyzing
human coprolites (30, 40) and of meticulously collecting
microfossils from habitation sites by flotation methods (37,
65), food remains from archaeological sites consisted mainly
of ossic materials that tended to be larger and better pre-
served. Remnants of phytic tissues, pollen, and other minute
organic debris were frequently overlooked.

Similarly, the few anthropologists who have made observations on the food habits of primitive groups have tended
to note the more visible and dramatic utilization of animal
food sources but have not accurately quantified the full
range of foods used. Nor has there been sufficient appre-
ciation of the extent of continuous foraging for plant products, which were usually ingested immediately wherever
gathered rather than being returned to the campsite (43, 50,
53, 54, 64, 67, 79). Reliance upon these biased sources of
dietary information has led frequently to the controversial,
if not erroneous, conclusion that early and preagricultural
human populations were dependent primarily upon animal,
rather than plant food sources (19, 39, 44, 82), despite
the fact that nearly all the higher primates are predominantly or exclusively herbivorous.

Technical refinements in the collection and analysis of
microfossils from soils uncovered in archaeological excavations (37, 58, 81), from intestinal contents of bogmen (32,
33) and desiccated corpses (81), and especially from extraordinarily well-preserved human coprolites (9 to 17, 22 to
25, 27, 28, 29 to 31, 40, 41, 45, 48, 49, 55, 58, 71, 73),
have increased greatly the data base available for recon-
struction of ancient human ecology. The wide variety of
known archaeological plant remains has been reviewed for both
the New World (60, 80) and the Middle East and Europe (51).
An annotated bibliography of publications on human coprolite
analysis has been published recently (74). One important
aspect of ancient human dietary practices now emerging from

the study of organic fossil materials painstakingly recovered
from human paleofeces is suggested by their incredibly high
content of undigested phytic remains (41). These most inti-
mate of ancient human artifacts, ignored or discarded during
many previous excavations, are providing the first direct
data confirming that at least some prehistoric populations
had learned to exploit and depend upon a wide variety of un-
cultivated plants as dietary staples to a degree heretofore
unrecognized.

II.   COPROLITES FROM PLEISTOCENE CONTEXTS

The emergence of several races of hominids is now
believed to have occurred at least 5 million years ago (70).
Fossil materials recovered from such early deposits are
fully mineralized and present technical problems to full
analysis which have yet to be overcome. Nevertheless,
Bonnefille (2) identified more than 50 types of pollen from
a supposed crocodile coprolite from the Omo Valley of
Ethiopia dated at more than 2.5 million years of age. Both
animal and probable human coprolites have been recovered
recently in association with early hominid skeletal remains
of similar age from the same general area (35, 38). Their
microfossil constituents have not been analyzed. Coprolite
specimens recovered from Olduvai Gorge in association with
Homo africanus remains dated at about 1 million years were
studied superficially by Napton (48) without notable success.
Imprints of seeds, leaves and stems, as well as whole endo-
carps of identifiable plants have been noted in coprolites
from the H. erectus deposits at Choukoutien in China (45).
Bryant and Williams-Dean (10) examined mineralized H. erectus
coprolites approximately 400,000 years of age from a European
site, the contents of which have not been fully characterized.
Coprolites believed to be those of H. sapiens neanderthalensis
examined by Callen (13) were found to contain bone remnants,
hair, charcoal, and other organic debris; pollen analysis was
not done.

As improved methods of thin-sectioning, scanning electron
microscopy, and techniques for dissolving mineralized specimens are developed, it is likely that much more information on
early hominid diets will become available.

III. DESICCATED COPROLITES FROM POSTPLEISTOCENE CONTEXTS

Desiccated, nonmineralized human coprolites from a variety of New World sites protected from moisture have proven to be most amenable to direct analysis, using the straightforward methods developed by Callen (16), Roust (55), and others. Investigators have analyzed dietary components from several comprehensive coprolite sequences, ranging in age from 500 to 10,000 years, recovered from sites in the American West (9, 17, 23, 25, 29), from Mammoth and Salts Caves in Kentucky (71, 72), and from sites in Central Mexico (11, 12, 14, 15), and Peru (15, 16). The evidence from these studies provides insight into the nature of early human dietary patterns which may have been the standard among hunter-gatherers over a time period several orders of magnitude greater than that directly represented by the data. Unfortunately, the significance of fibrous constituents was not recognized, and quantitative measurements of the various plant tissues from these coprolites have been reported only occasionally in the literature. While the phytic remains generally were separated into seeds, achenes, stalks, leaves, epidermis, pericarps, etc., percentage weights of each component relative to the original weight of dry sample have been recorded from only three sites: Lovelock and Hidden Caves, Nevada (17, 55), Hogup Cave, Utah (25), and Mammoth and Salts Caves, Kentucky (63).

From the published data on these three series of human coprolites, one can derive approximate mean values for the percentage content of undigested plant fiber residue on a dry-weight basis for comparison with contemporary populations on various dietary regimes.

Samples of whole or incomplete paleofecal specimens either were picked apart carefully in the dry state or soaked for several days in 0.2 percent trisodium phosphate and passed through graded screens before separation of macrofossil constituents. Pollen grains, a major constituent of some specimens, can be collected by several sedimentation/flotation techniques (10, 49, 58). Fibrous residues ranged in maximum diameter from small pieces of masticated leaves and stalks (<2 mm), seeds and achenes (1 to 2 mm), down to a fine, paperlike mesh of fibrils (<0.5 mm) which coated the 350-μ screens in many samples (Figure 2). As the chemical nature of each constituent was not determined in any of the

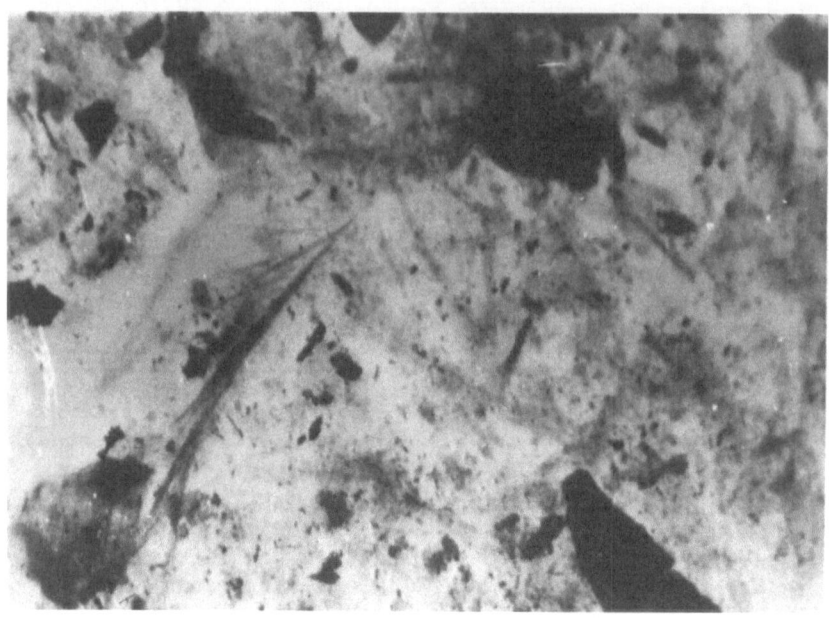

Figure 2. Amorphous, paperlike fibrous mesh retained on
350-μ screens during separation of coprolite constituents;
Lovelock Cave. Fragments of bones, seeds, achenes, microfibrils, and minute feather parts are seen. X50
(reduced 30% for reproduction).

studies, all plant products are lumped together as fiber
residues for ease of calculation.

    The most extensive series of coprolite analyses have
been made by R. F. Heizer and colleagues at the University
of California, Berkeley, on specimens derived from Lovelock
Cave and several nearby Great Basin sites. Analysis of over
600 of the several thousand specimens recovered clearly revealed a stable, lacustrine subsistence pattern based on
plant and small-animal resources available around the immediate lakeshore and adjacent desertic habitats (29, 30, 31).
The fiber residue content of a large series of these specimens was 25 to 34% (30%) of original dry weight (41). Intact
seeds and ground, cracked, or parched achenes accounted for
50 to 70% of the total fibrous residue, of which those of
the common tule or bulrush (Scirpus sp.) predominated

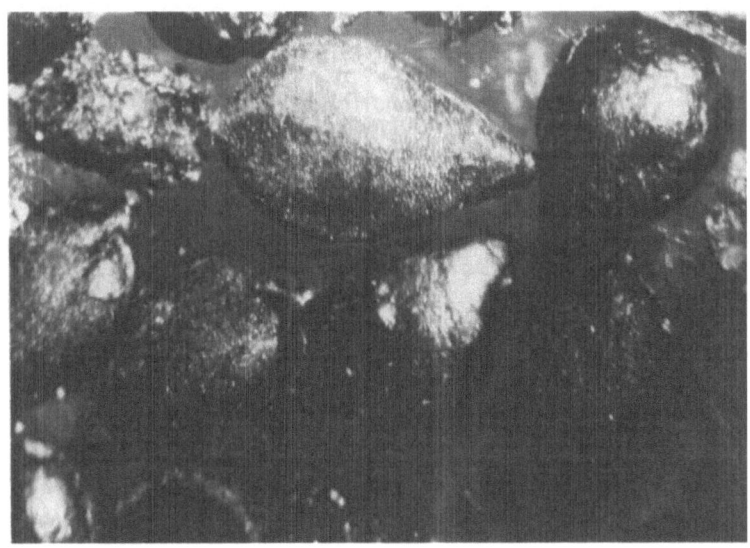

Figure 3a. Seeds and seed fragments recovered from a Lovelock Cave coprolite. <u>Scirpus</u> sp. (tuleweed or bulrush). X20.

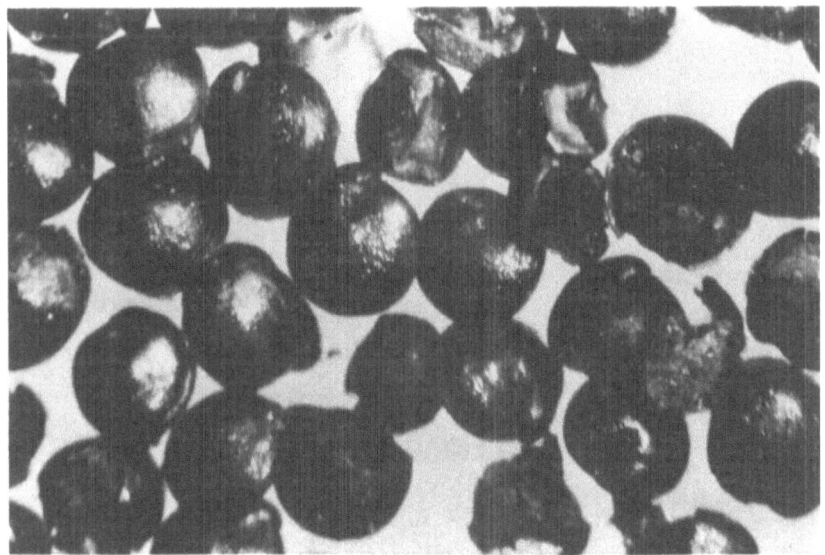

Figure 3b. Seeds and seed fragments recovered from a Lovelock Cave coprolite. <u>Suaeda depressa</u> (saltbush). X40
(both reduced 35% for reproduction).

(Figure 3). An additional 2 to 17% of the total fibrous
residue, particularly amid the fine, paperlike mesh, were
derived principally from the stalks of the tule and cattail
(Typha sp.). Several thousand discarded "quids," consisting
of the masticated stalks of these plants, have been recovered
(Figure 4). One 58-g coprolite specimen contained nearly
90% cattail pollen. Seeds, epidermis, pericarps, and other
tissues of a chenopod (Suaeda depressa) (Figure 2), panic
grass (Panicum sp.), wild flax (Linum sp.), arrowcane
(Phragmites sp.), and squaw grass (Elymus sp.) were recovered in lesser frequency (30). Two specimens analyzed
for total cellulose using ether extraction and chromatographic techniques yielded values of 23.8% and 33.8% (48).
Faunal components, consisting mostly of flesh and the bones
and scales of small fish (22,23) and bones and feathers or
hair of birds and rodents, constituted 9 to 12% (10%) of
the dietary remnants recovered (Figure 5).

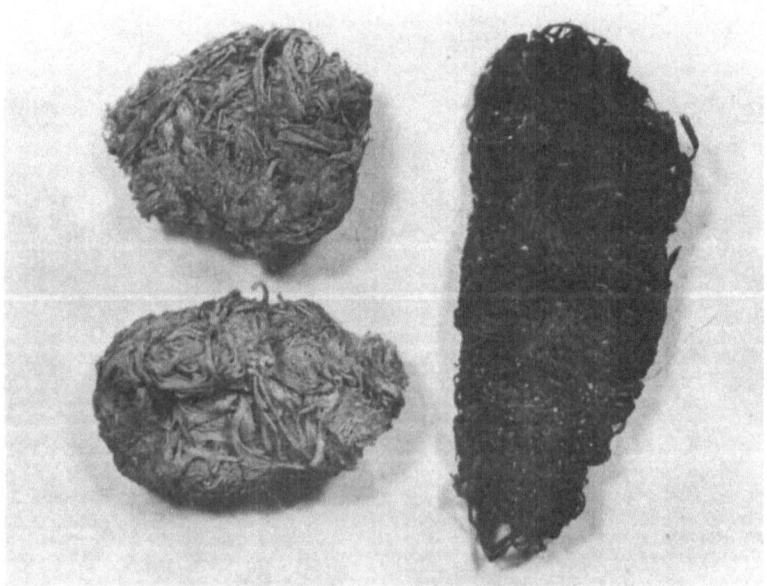

Figure 4. Masticated quids of tuleweed stalks discarded in
Lovelock Cave; probably source of much of amorphous fibrous
remains in coprolites. X2 (reduced 25% for reproduction).

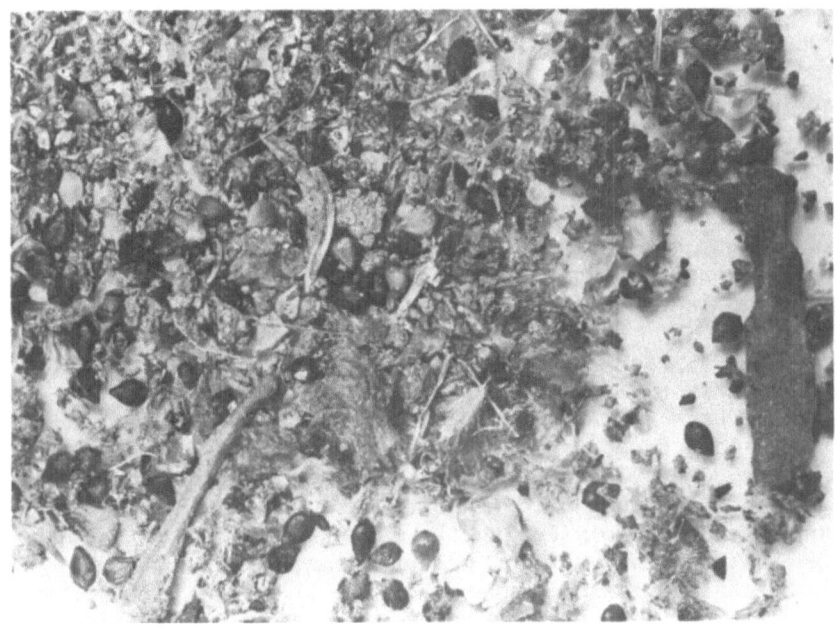

Figure 5. Unseparated dried residues from Lovelock Cave
coprolite after reconstitution and screening: fish bones,
duck feathers, and Scirpus seeds predominate. Note some
seeds are a natural light (brown) color, while most are
blackened from parching or baking prior to ingestion. X2
(reduced 25% for reproduction).

     Analysis of coprolites from an ecologically similar
riparian site in the desert of the American West has
revealed a similar dependence on plant food sources and a
comparable content of undigested phytic remains. Based on
30 specimens from Hogup Cave in Utah, Fry (24, 25) has
described a subsistence regime based on the utilization of
the seeds of a chenopod, pickleweed, or burroweed (Allenrolfea occidentalis), and various tissues of the prickly
pear cactus (Opuntia sp.). Total seed residues of these
specimens ranged from 11.3 to 22.3% of original dry weight;
Opuntia tissues accounted for 1.3 to 11.9%, and unidentified
plant epidermis, stems, and fibers for an additional 16.8 to
29.1%. Overall, combined phytic remains accounted for 43 to
50% (46%) of the original dry weight of the specimens examined (41). Bone and other faunal remnants constituted about
2 to 8% of the paleofecal contents.

Several cultural horizons, dating back to at least
9000 B.C., are discernible in the excavations of Danger
and Hogup caves. An increasing dietary dependence upon
grasses rather than Allenrolfea is evident in the more
recent materials of post-1000 B.C. Several specimens were
found to "contain large amounts of finely chopped shrub
stems that are undoubtedly herbivore browse. Thus, it
appears probable that some of the members of the prehistoric society ate the stomach contents of large herbivores"
(25), a practice which has been verified by ethnographic
observations.

Dietary data from a series of carefully controlled
excavations and analyses at the Mammoth and Salts caves
complex have recently been published by Watson (71, 72)
and associates (58, 63, 73, 81). Again, a chenopod
species, Chenopodium hybridum, together with sunflower
(Helianthus annuus), formed the basis of abroadly phytic
subsistence economy during the Early Woodland horizon of
the last millennium B.C. Calculations based on the constituent analysis of Stewart (63) on 11 of the Salts Cave
coprolites indicated that plant fiber residues constituted
34 to 90% (58%) of the original dry weight of the samples,
while faunal remains, when present, ranged from 4 to 40%
(9%). Other plant debris found in significant quantities
included hickory nutshells, squash tissues and grape seeds.

Findings from analysis of coprolites from Texas rock-
shelter sites (9), Clydes Cavern (76), Ocampo Caves and
Tehuacan in Mexico (11 to 14) and Huaca Prieta in Peru (16)
appear to support the conclusion that preagricultural human
populations in these areas ingested large quantities of
coarse plant materials. That these dietary patterns per-
sisted for at least 10,000 years is established; indeed,
they may well indicate the nature of hominoid diets over
truly evolutionary time periods.

Despite the well-documented laxative effects of diets
high in cellulose and hemicellulose residues (18, 21, 75),
constipation and difficulty in evacuating these incredibly
coarse, bone-studded "fecal pellets...sometimes three inches
in diameter...so solid and packed with fiber and seeds that
they can only have been passed with great effort" (29) must
have been more than an occasional problem in these prehistoric populations. Ethnobotanical accounts among several

Great Basin Indian populations, presumably descendant from
the paleo-Indians whose coprolites have been studied, reveal
that a wide variety of cathartic, emetic, and laxative
plant substances were in common use (68). Similarly, among
the salts known to have been mined by the prehistoric Salts
Cavers were abudant deposits of mirabilite ($Na_2SO_4 \cdot 10H_2O$),
presumably for its powerful cathartic properties (73).
Knowledge of such substances (69) and, indeed, the well-
documented use of native bladder and reed enemata was wide-
spread throughout the Americas (28). It is possible that
excessive doses of plant fiber in the diet, particularly
lignin, may have been responsible for causing considerable
constipation, as is suggested by the recent studies of Harvey
et al. (27) on the contradictory effects of high-residue diets
in contemporary human subjects.

In order to approach a rough estimate of the fiber content of coprolites on a wet-weight basis, three complete
and intact Lovelock Cave specimens were selected for total
rehydration in sealed bell jars over a solution mixed from
equal parts of 0.5% trisodium phosphate:95% alcohol:10% for-
malin and maintained in an incubator at 34°C for several
months (41). Following this treatment, the three specimens
exhibited a 98% mean increase in weight and averaged 220 g
in final wet weight, which is comparable to stool weights
reported by Burkitt (5) for African villagers on a traditional, high-residue diet. Assuming that on the average,
at least 50% of the ingested plant fiber is digested in
passage (62, 75), and given a mean coprolite fiber content
of 30%, approximately 130 g of plant fiber would have been
ingested to produce the stools observed. The daily dietary
fiber intake of contemporary urban adults has been estimated
to range between 16 to 28 g (United Kingdom) and 20 to 30 g
(United States) (18). However, without knowledge of transit
time and total daily fecal output, estimates of daily dietary
fiber intake cannot be made with any great accuracy for prehistoric populations.

In postneolithic Europe, discoveries of cached food
supplies (51) and the recovery of intestinal content of bogmen (32, 33) indicate that despite the introduction of
domesticated cereal grains, coarse, wild seed crops continued to be an important source of food in the period from
7000 to 1000 B.C. The fiber content of the various wild
seed crops utilized in both the New World and Europe in

prehistoric times ranged from 12 to 30%, while domesticated
cereal grains (wheat, oats, maize, and barley) range from
1 to 3% (77). Based on the nature of the primary cereal
crops utilized during the past 15,000 years, the human diet
in the Old World as well as the New has apparently undergone
several identifiable revolutions (Figure 1). The net result
of this process of domestication and refinement of primary
food sources has been a decrease in dietary fiber content by
approximately 90%. The replacement of a considerable portion
of foraged seed grains by primitive Emmer wheat alone resulted
in a 50% decrease in cereal fiber content.

IV. THE ROLE OF NONPHYTIC BIOPOLYMERS
IN PREAGRICULTURAL HUMAN DIETS

In the three New World coprolite populations discussed
above for which adequate data were available, phytic materials constituted the greater part of undigested residues.
Significant, often spectacular, quantities of animal tissues
in the form of bones, teeth, feathers, hair, keratinized skin,
fish scales, and insect cuticle frequently contributed more
than 10% of the total weight of undigested residues. In
some specimens, the remains of dozens of small fish out-
weighed the plant residues (22, 23). While the primary
focus of this discussion is upon the functions and effects
of ingested plant tissues, it must be kept in mind that such
undigestible animal tissues are also biopolymers and potentially capable of some of the same physiological functions
in human nutrition as cellulose, hemicellulose, and lignin.
Furthermore, as modern man no longer ingests whole birds,
rodents, reptiles, and insects, these particular biopolymers
were not merely reduced in quantity but were totally elimi-
nated from the diet. Hydroxyapatite of bone, keratin of
skin, feathers, scales, etc., and acetylglucosamine and
scleratin of insect cuticle may be regarded as the zootic
counterparts of cellulose, hemicellulose, and lignin, in
that they provide a matrix for binding protein and strength-
ening the architecture of the organism. Thus, they may play
similar roles in the digestive and excretory processes when
ingested as food.

V. POSSIBLE MORPHOLOGICAL ADAPTATIONS TO THE
FIBER CONTENT OF THE DIET

Numerous desiccated, frozen, or mummified human corpses
have been recovered from postpleistocene archeological sites.
Even under the best conditions of preservation, however,
details of morphology and histology have not proven to be
amenable to study. Materials from earlier, Pleistocene
deposits consist entirely of mineralized hard tissues or,
rarely, casts of some of the internal organs. Therefore,
in discussing possible adaptive changes in response to diet,
one can only extrapolate from the physical nature of the
presumed diet and the structure, function and dysfunction
of the digestive organs in man and the herbivorous pongid
primates to arrive, albeit teleologically, at some conclusions.

The presence throughout the intestine, in both chimpanzee (4, 61) and man, of a well-developed circular and
longitudinal muscularis externa designed to actively propel
a fairly large, soft fecal bolus might be interpreted as an
evolutionary response to countless generations of exposure
to a high-residue diet. Likewise, the presence of saccula-
tions (haustra) in the large intestine provide increased
surface area for the rapid endogenous and bacterial enzymatic
extraction of nutrients from large quantities of plant tissues. Among the strictly herbivorous pongid primates, increased sacculation and numerous functional appendices of
the cecum allow for the efficient digestion of plant tissues
by bacterial processes. The vermiform appendix in contemporary man has become too short and narrow to allow its
proper digestive function, probably as a direct result of
10,000 years of selective pressure by low-residue diets and
acute disease caused by atrophic occlusion.

Recent studies indicate that low-residue diets cause
alterations in the intestinal flora in humans (20). Shaedler
(56) found that low-residue diets in rodents decreased the
density of the intestinal flora and in germ-free animals,
decreased peristalsis, increased transit time and resulted
in an enlarged, thin-walled cecum, perhaps a result of the
effects of an "endogenous hypertensive enzyme...a kinin-
releasing protease...characterized by trypsin."

In general, one might hypothesize that, other than the
reduction in size of the vermiform appendix, no significant
morphological adaptive changes have occurred in the human
gastrointestinal tract as a result of the increasing refinement of the diet. Selection pressures would not be likely
to effect phenotypic changes toward low-fiber adaptation, as
disease entities believed to be related to dietary fiber
deficiencies are chronic, slow-developing disabilities,
occurring mostly in the postprocreative decades. Function-
ally, however, in individuals existing on highly refined
diets, the chronic lack (3) of sufficient bulk to fill the
intestinal lumen and stimulate peristalsis would be expected
to decrease tonus in the muscularis externa, leading to atrophy and potential herniation of the intestinal wall. This
hypothesis might be suitably tested in the laboratory by
comparing the functional anatomy of chimpanzees on long-term
dietary regimes of varying levels of fiber residue. In the
absence of sufficient data on experimental, anatomical and
field studies of the normal as well as pathological range of
pognid gastroenterology and dietetics, even these hypotheses
must be regarded as highly speculative.

VI. SUMMARY

The role of dietary fiber in the preagricultural subsistence economy of early human populations strongly suggests
that for over 99% of man's existence as a distinct species,
his gastrointestinal tract has been exposed to the selective
pressures exerted by a coarse, high-residue diet of plant
tissues. While lower Pleistocene human coprolites have not
yet proved amenable to study, analyses of several large
series of desiccated paleofecal specimens covering time spans
of up to 10,000 years have revealed that undigested plant tissues account for 30 to 50% of the dry weight of the stool.
Coprolite rehydration experiments indicate that roughly 130 g
of plant tissues would have been ingested to account for the
residues present in a single, whole stool specimen. Coprolite studies also suggest a possible physiological role for
nonphytic biopolymers such as those resulting from the ingestion of entire uncooked fish, birds, reptiles, small mammals,
and insects.

It is hypothesized that dependence on a broadly based,
highly phytic dietary regime remained rather constant for
several millions of years until the advent of agriculture and

the introduction of domesticated cereal grains approximately
15,000 to 20,000 years ago. Alterations in the physiology
of the gastrointestinal tract arising since that advance
(with the possible exception of the atrophy of the vermiform appendix) would be expected to be of a functional
(ontogenous) rather than a morphological (phylogenous) nature.

REFERENCES

1. Anderson, R. D., Calvo, J., Serrano, G., and Payne,
    G. C., 1946, A study of the nutritional status and
    food habits of Otomi Indians in the Mezquital Valley
    of Mexico, Am. J. Pub. Hlth., 36:833.

2. Boeles, J. J., 1963, Second expedition to the Mrabri
    of North Thailand ("Khon Pa"), J. Siam. Soc., 51:133.

3. Bonnefille, R., 1970, Premiers resultats convernant
    l'analyse pollinique d'echantillons due Pleistocene
    inferieur de l'Omo (Ethiope), C. R. Acad. Sci., 270:2430.

4. Bourne, G. H., editor, The Chimpanzee, Vol. 5, Histol-
    ogy and Reproduction and Restraint (New York:S. Karger,
    1970).

5. Burkitt, D. P., 1973, Some diseases characteristic of
    Western civilization, Brit. Med. J., 3:274.

6. Burkitt, D. P., Walker, A. R. P., and Painter, N. S.,
    1974, Dietary fiber and disease, J. Am. Med. Assoc.,
    229:1068.

7. Briggs, G., and Lang, J., "The use and function of
    fiber for diets for monogastric experimental animals,"
    in: Fibers in Human Nutrition, edited by G. S. Spiller
    and R. J. Amen (Springfield: C. C. Thomas, 1976).

8. Bryant, V. M., 1974, The role of coprolite analysis
    in archeology, Bull. Texas Archeol. Soc., 45:1.

9. Bryant, V. M., 1974, Prehistoric diet in southwest
    Texas: the coprolite evidence, Amer. Antiq., 39:407.

10. Bryant, V. M., and Williams-Dean, G., 1975, The copro-
     lites of man, Sci. Am., 232:100.

11. Callen, E. O., "Analysis of the Tehuacan coprolites,"
     in: The Prehistory of the Tehuacan Valley, Vol. 1,
     Environment and Subsistence, edited by D. S. Byers
     (Austin: University of Texas Press, 1967), p. 261.

12. Callen, E. O., Plants, diet and early agriculture of
     some cave-dwelling pre-Colombian Mexican Indians,
     Actas y Memorias 37th Congr. Int. Americanistas,
     II:641 (Buenos Aires) 1968.

13. Callen, E. O., 1969, Les coprolithes de la cabane
     acheuleene du Lazart: Analyse et Diagnostic., Mem.
     Soc. Prehist. Francaise, 7:123.

14. Callen, E. O., "Dietary patterns in Mexico between
     6500 B. C. and 1580 A. D.," in: Man and His Foods,
     edited by C. Earle Smith (University of Alabama:
     University of Alabama Press, 1969).

15. Callen, E. O., "Diet as revealed in coprolites," in:
     Science in Archaeology, edited by D. Brothwell and
     E. S. Higgs (New York: Praeger Publishers, 1970).

16. Callen, E. O., and Cameron, T. W. M., 1960, A prehis-
     toric diet revealed in coprolites, The New Scientist,
     8:35.

17. Cowan, R. A., 1967, Lake margin ecologic exploitation
     in the Great Basin as demonstrated by an analysis of
     coprolites from Lovelock Cave, Nevada, Report U. C.
     (Berkeley) Archaeol. Survey, 70:21.

18. Cummings, J. H., 1974, Progress report. Dietary fiber,
     Gut, 14:69.

19. Dornstreich, M. D., 1973, Food habits of early man:
     balance between hunting and gathering, Science, 179:306.

20. Drasar, B. S., Crowther, J. S., Goddard, P., Hawksworth,
     G., Hill, M. J., Peach, S., Williams, R. E., and Renwich,
     A., 1973, The relation between diet and the gut micro-
     flora in man, Proc. Nutr. Soc., 32:49.

21.   Eastwood, M. A., 1974, Dietary fiber in human nutrition,
      J. Sci. Fd. Agric., 25:1523.

22.   Follett, W. I., 1967, Fish remains from coprolites and
      midden deposits at Lovelock Cave, Churchill County,
      Nevada, report U. C. (Berkeley) Archaeol. Survey,
      70:93.

23.   Follett, W. I., 1970, Fish remains from human coprolites
      and midden deposits obtained during 1968 and 1969 at
      Lovelock Cave, Churchill County, Nevada, Contr. U. C.
      (Berkeley) Archaeol. Research Facility, 10:163.

24.   Fry, G. F., 1970, Prehistoric human ecology in Utah;
      based on the analysis of coprolites, Ph.D. thesis,
      Univ. of Utah, Department of Anthropology.

25.   Fry, G. F., 1970,"Preliminary analysis of the Hogup
      Cave coprolites," in: Hogup Cave, University of Utah
      Anthrop. Paper No. 93.

26.   Goodall, J., "Chimpanzees of the Gombe Stream Reserve,"
      in: Primate Behavior, edited by I. DeVore (New York:
      Holt, Rinehart & Winston, 1965).

27.   Harvey, R. F., Pomare, E. W. and Heaton, K. W., Effects
      of increased dietary fiber on intestinal transit,
      Lancet, 1:1278.

28.   Heizer, R. F., 1939, The bulbed enema syringe and enema
      tube in the New World, Primitive Man, 12:85.

29.   Heizer, R. F., "The anthropology of prehistoric Great
      Basin human coprolites," in: Science and Archaeology,
      edited by D. Brothwell and E. S. Higgs (New York:
      Praeger Publishers, 1970).

30.   Heizer, R. F., and Napton, L. K., 1969, Biological
      and cultural evidence from prehistoric human copro-
      lites, Science, 165:563.

31.   Heizer, R. F., and Napton, L. K., 1970, Archaeology and
      the prehistoric Great Basin lacustrine subsistence
      regime as seen from Lovelock Cave, Nevada, Contr. U. C.
      (Berkeley) Archaeol. Research Facility, 10:1.

32. Helbaek, H., 1958, Grauballe mandens sidste Maltid.
    Kuml: Arbog for Jysk Arkaeologisk Selskan, Copenhagen.

33. Helbaek, H., "Paleoethnobotany," in: Science and
    Archaeology, edited by D. Brothwell and E. S. Higgs
    (New York: Praeger Publishers, 1970).

34. Hightower, N. C., and Janowitz, H. D., "Digestion,"
    in: Physiological Basis of Medical Practice, edited
    by Best and Taylor (Baltimore: Williams and Williams
    Co., 1973).

35. Howell, F. C., personal communication.

36. Hungate, R. E., "Microbial activities related to mam-
    malian digestion and absorption of food," in: Fiber
    in Human Nutrition, edited by G. A. Spiller and R. J.
    Amen (Springfield: C. C. Thomas, 1976).

37. Jarman, H. N., Legge, A. J., and Charles, J. A., "Re-
    trieval of plant remains from archaeological sites by
    froth flotation," in: Papers in Economic Prehistory,
    edited by E. S. Higgs (London: Cambridge University
    Press, 1972) p. 39.

38. Johanson, D. C., personal communication.

39. Jolly, C. J., The seed eaters: A new model of hominid
    differentiation based on a baboon analogy, Man, March
    1970.

40. Jones, V. H., "The vegetal remains of Newt Cash Hollow
    Shelter," in: Rock Shelters of Menifee County, Kentucky,
    edited by W. S. Webb and W. D. Funkhouser (Lexington:
    University of Kentucky, 1936) Reports in Archaeology
    and Ethnology, 3:147.

41. Kliks, M., Paleoepidemiological studies on Great Basin
    coprolites: estimation of dietary fiber intake and
    evaluation of the ingestion of anthelmintic plant sub-
    stances, Contr. U.C. (Berkeley) Archaeol. Research
    Facility, in press, 1975.

42. Leaky, M. D., Olduvai Gorge: Excavations in Beds I and
    II, 1960-1963 (London: Cambridge University Press), 1971.

43. Lee, R. B., "What hunters do for a living, or how to make out on scarce resources," in: Man the Hunter, R. B. Lee and I. DeVore, editors (Chicago: Aldine, 1968).

44. Leopold, A. C., and Ardrey, R., 1972, Toxic substances in plants and the food habits of early man, Science, 176:512.

45. Li Yiu-Heng, et al., 1966, Preliminary observations on some coprolites from Choukoutien, Vertebrate Palasiatica, 10:73.

46. McClure, H. E., 1964, Some observations of primates in climax dipterocarp forest near Kuala Lumpur, Malaysia, Primates, 5:39.

47. Metz, J., Hart, D., and Harpending, H. C., 1971, Iron, folate and vitamin B_{12} in a hunter-gatherer people: a study of the Kung Bushmen, Am. J. Clin. Nutr., 24:229.

48. Napton, L. K., and Heizer, R. F., 1970, Analyses of human coprolites from archaeological contexts with primary reference to Lovelock Cave, Nevada, Contr. U.C. (Berkeley) Archaeol. Research Facility, 10:87.

49. Napton, L. K., Heizer, R. F., and Kelso, G., "Preliminary palynological analysis of Lovelock Cave coprolites," in: Archaeological and Paleobiological Investigation in Lovelock Cave, Nevada, Kroeber Anthropological Society, Special Publication No. 2, Berkeley, 1969.

50. Quinn, P. J., Foods and Feeding Habits of the Pedi (Johannesburg: Withwatersrand University Press, 1959).

51. Renfrew, J. M., Paleoenthnobotany: The Prehistoric Food Plants of the Near East and Europe (New York: Columbia University Press, 1973).

52. Reynolds, V., and Reynolds, F., "Chimpanzees in the Budongo Forest," in: Primate Behavior, I. DeVore, editor (New York: Holt, Rinehart & Winston, 1965) p. 368.

53. Richards, A. I., Hunger and Work in a Savage Tribe: A Functional Study of Nutrition Among the Southern Bantu (London: G. Routledge & Sons, Ltd., 1932).

54. Roth, W. E., 1901, Food, its search, capture and pre-
    paration, North Queensland Ethnog. Bull. No. 3, p. 1.

55. Roust, N. L., 1970, Preliminary examination of pre-
    historic human coprolites from four western Nevada
    caves, Report U.C. Archaeol. Survey, 70:49.

56. Schaedler, R. W., 1973, Symposium on gut microflora
    and nutrition in the nonruminant. The relationship
    between the host and its intestinal microflora, Proc.
    Nutr. Soc., 32:41.

57. Schaller, G., "The mountain gorilla: ecology and be-
    havior," in: Primate Behavior, I. DeVore, editor (New
    York: Holt, Rinehart & Winston, 1965) p. 324.

58. Schoenwetter, J., "Pollen analysis of human paleofeces
    from Upper Salts Cave," in: The Archaeology of the
    Mammoth Cave Area, P. J. Watson, editor (New York:
    Academic Press, 1974).

59. Schdder, T., 1971, Gathering among African woodland
    savannah cultivators, a case study: the Gwembe Tonga,
    Zambian Papers, 5.

60. Smith, C. E., Callen, E. O., Cutler, H. C., Galinat,
    W. C., Kaplan, L., Witaker, T. W., and Yarnell, R. A.,
    1966, Bibliography of American archaeological plant
    remains, Econ. Bot., 20:446.

61. Sonntag, C. F., 1923, The anatomy, physiology and path-
    ology of the chimpanzee, Proc. Zool. Soc., p. 323.

62. Southgate, D. A. T., and Durnin, J. V. G. A., 1970,
    Calorie conversion factors. An experimental reassess-
    ment of the factors used in the calculation of the energy
    value of human diets, Brit. J. Nutr., 24:517.

63. Stewart, R. B., "Identification and quantification of
    components in Salts Cave paleofeces, 1970-1972," in:
    The Archaeology of the Mammoth Cave Area, P. J. Watson,
    editor (New York: Academic Press, 1974).

64. Story, R., 1958, Some plants used by the Bushmen in ob-
    taining food and water, Botanical Survey Memoir No. 30,
    Dept. of Agriculture, Div. of Botany, Pretoria.

65. Streuver, S., 1968, Flotation techniques for the re-
    covery of small-scale archaeological remains, Amer.
    Anthrop., 33:353.

66. Suzuki, A., 1969, An ecological study of chimpanzees in
    a savanna woodland, Primates, 10:103.

67. Tomita, K., 1966, The sources of food for the Hadzapi
    tribe: The life of a hunting tribe in East Africa,
    Kyoto Univ. African Studies, 1:157.

68. Train, P., Henrichs, J. R., and Archer, W. A., 1957,
    Medicinal uses of plants by the Indian tribes of Nevada.
    Contributions toward a flora of Nevada, No. 45, U.S.
    Natl. Arboretum, U.S. Dept. of Agriculture, Washington,
    D.C.

69. Vogel, V. J., American Indian Medicine (Norman: Univ.
    of Oklahoma Press, 1970).

70. Washburn, S. L., and Moore, R., Ape Into Man: A Study
    of Human Evolution (Boston: Little, Brown and Co., 1974).

71. Watson, P. J., 1969, The prehistory of Salts Cave, Ken-
    tucky, III. State Museum Reports of Investigations
    No. 16, Springfield.

72. Watson, P. J., editor, The Archeology of the Mammoth
    Cave Area (New York: Academic Press, 1974).

73. Watson, P. J., and Yarnell, R. A., 1966, Archaeological
    and Paleoethnobotanical investigations in Salts Cave,
    Mammoth Cave National Park, Kentucky, Amer. Antiq.,
    31:842.

74. Wilke, P. J., and Hall, H. J., Analysis of ancient
    feces: A descriptive bibliography, Contr. U.C. (Berkeley)
    Archaeol. Research Facility, in press, 1975.

75. Williams, R. D., and Olmstead, W. H., 1936, The manner
    in which food controls the bulk of the feces, Ann. Int.
    Med., 10:717.

76. Winter, J. C., and Wylie, H. G., 1974, Paleoecology and
    diet at Clydes Cavern, Amer. Antiq., 39:305.

77. Winton, A. L., and Winton, K. B., The Structure and
    Composition of Foods, Vol. 1. Cereals, Starch, Oil
    Seeds, Nuts, Oils, Forage Plants (New York: John Wiley),
    1932).

78. Winton, M., 1970, Nutritional adaptation of some Colom-
    bian Indians, Am. J. Phys. Anthrop., 32:293.

79. Woodburn, J., "An introduction to Hadza ecology," in:
    Man the Hunter, R. B. Lee and I. DeVore, editors
    (Chicago: Aldine, 1968).

80. Yarnell, R. A., "Paleoethnobotany in America," in:
    Science in Archaeology, D. Brothwell and E. S. Higgs,
    editors (New York: Praeger Publishers, 1970) p. 215.

81. Yarnell, R. A., "Intestinal contents of the Salts Cave
    mummy and analysis of the initial Salts Cave flotation
    series," in: The Archeology of the Mammoth Cave Area,
    P. J. Watson, editor (New York: Academic Press, 1974).

82. Yudkin, J., "Archaeology and the nutritionist," in:
    The Domestication and Exploitation of Plants and Ani-
    mals, P. J. Ucko and G. W. Dimleby, editors, (Chicago:
    Aldine, 1969).

APPENDIX

DIETARY FIBER CONTENT OF FOODS

Elizabeth A. Shipley

Department of Nutritional Science
Syntex Research

Palo Alto, California

The increasing interest in dietary fiber and its relation to human health and disease (4, 7) has created a great
need for food composition tables that give the dietary fiber
content of foods.

The biggest obstacle to the development of such tables
has been the lack of agreement among investigators on which
plant polymers to include in the definition of dietary fiber
and what to call the sum of the individual components. For-
tunately, most investigators now agree that dietary fiber is
the sum of all plant polysaccharides (cellulose, hemicelluloses, pectins, gums, and mucilages) plus lignin that are
not digested by human digestive enzymes (but not excluding
possible digestion by colonic microflora). Several terms
have been suggested for the sum of these various components,
including "dietary fiber," "unavailable carbohydrate," and
"indigestible residue," dietary fiber being the best known.
Because "fiber" is an inexact word, used in many other fields,
Spiller et al. (6) have recently suggested "plantix" as an
alternate term.

Other impediments to the development of food tables
that include the dietary fiber (plantix) content of foods
have been the lack of precise analytical methodologies
and disagreement on how to present the data. At the present
time, most food composition tables either do not include
values for dietary fiber (plantix) or use crude fiber values
to represent dietary fiber (plantix) content of foods. How-

ever, crude fiber values greatly underestimate the total
dietary fiber (plantix) content of foods because a large
percentage of the cellulose, hemicelluloses and lignins
and all of the pectins, gums and mucilages are lost in
the analyses. Food tables that give both the total dietary
fiber (plantix) content of foods and the percent contribution of each individual component (i.e., cellulose, hemicelluloses, lignins, pectins, gums and mucilages) would
undoubtedly be of the greatest value.

It is hoped that in the near future universal agreement will be reached on the definition, nomenclature,
analysis and presentation of analyses of dietary fiber
(plantix) so that the work of different investigators may
be easily compared.

The purpose of this appendix is to provide dietary
fiber (plantix) values for use by nutritionists and dieti-
cians. The following tables are a compilation of the dietary fiber (plantix) values or fractions thereof available
at the present time. The values presented represent the
work of several investigators and, as a result, both the
analytical method used in the determination and the term
applied to the dietary fraction analyzed vary with investigators.

Table 1 gives dietary fiber (plantix) values as determined by the Southgate methodology (2). Table 2 compares
the Van Soest NDF methodology (4) with the Hellendoorn
enzymatic methodology (1), neither of which includes pectins,
water-soluble gums or mucilages in the determination.

TABLE 1. Dietary Fiber (Plantix) Content of Various Foods

(g/100 g edible portion)

Food	Crude fiber[1]	Total Dietary fiber (Plantix)[2]	Noncellulosic Polysaccharides[2]	Cellulose[2]	Lignin[2]
Grains and grain products					
Flour, white	0.30	3.15	2.52	0.60	0.03
Flour, whole-wheat	2.30	9.51	6.25	2.46	0.80
Bran	9.41	44.00	32.70	8.05	3.23
Bread, white	0.20	2.72	2.01	0.71	tr
Bread, whole-wheat	1.60	8.50	5.95	1.31	1.24
All-Bran®	7.80	26.70	17.82	6.01	2.88
Cornflakes	0.70	11.00	7.26	2.42	1.32
Grape-Nuts®	–	7.00	5.14	1.28	0.58
Rice Krispies®	0.60	4.47	3.47	0.78	0.22
Puffed Wheat®	2.00	15.41	10.35	2.59	2.47
Sugar Puffs®	0.30	6.08	4.00	0.99	1.09
Shredded Wheat®	2.30	12.26	8.79	2.63	0.84
Special K®	–	5.45	3.68	0.72	1.05
Fruits					
Apples, flesh only	0.60	1.42	0.94	0.48	0.01
Apples, peel only	0.40	3.71	2.21	1.01	0.49
Bananas	0.50	1.75	1.12	0.37	0.26
Cherries, flesh & skin	0.40	1.24	0.92	0.25	0.07

TABLE 1. Dietary Fiber (Plantix) Content of Various Foods (Continued)

(g/100 g edible portion)

Food	Crude fiber[1]	Total Dietary fiber (Plantix)[2]	Noncellulosic Polysaccharides[2]	Cellulose[2]	Lignin[2]
Fruits, continued					
Grapefruit, cnd	0.40	0.44	0.34	0.04	0.55
Guavas, cnd	5.64 (raw)	3.64	1.67	1.17	0.80
Mandarin oranges, cnd	0.50 (raw)	0.29	0.22	0.04	0.03
Mangoes, cnd	0.90 (raw)	1.00	0.65	0.32	0.03
Peaches, flesh & skin	0.60	2.28	1.46	0.20	0.62
Pears, flesh only	} 1.40	2.44	1.32	0.67	0.45
Pears, peel only		8.59	3.72	2.18	2.67
Plums, flesh & skin	0.50	1.52	0.99	0.23	0.30
Rhubarb, raw	0.70	1.78	0.93	0.70	0.15
Strawberries, raw	1.30	2.12	0.98	0.33	0.81
Strawberries, cnd	0.60	1.00	0.48	0.20	0.33
Nuts and nut products					
Brazil	3.10	7.73	3.60	2.17	1.96
Peanuts	2.04	9.30	6.40	1.69	1.21
Peanut butter	1.90	7.55	5.64	1.91	tr
Vegetables					
Beans, baked	1.50	7.27	5.67	1.41	0.19
Beans, green	1.00	3.35	1.85	1.29	0.21
Broccoli, ckd	1.50	4.10	2.92	0.85	0.03
Brussel sprouts, ckd	1.60	2.86	1.99	0.80	0.07

TABLE 1. Dietary Fiber (Plantix) Content of Various Foods (Continued)

(g/100 g edible portion)

Food	Crude fiber[1]	Total Dietary fiber (Plantix)[2]	Noncellulosic Polysaccharides[2]	Cellulose[2]	Lignin[2]
Vegetables, continued					
Cabbage, ckd	0.80	2.83	1.76	0.69	0.38
Carrots, ckd	1.00	3.70	2.22	1.48	tr
Cauliflower, ckd	1.00	1.80	0.67	1.13	tr
Corn, sweet, ckd	0.70	4.74	4.31	0.31	0.12
Corn, sweet, cnd	0.80	5.69	4.97	0.64	0.08
Lettuce, raw	0.60	1.53	0.47	1.06	tr
Onions, raw	0.60	2.10	1.55	0.55	tr
Parsnips, raw	2.00	4.90	3.77	1.13	tr
Peas, frozen, raw	1.90	7.75	5.48	2.09	0.18
Peas, cnd	1.40	7.07	4.50	2.39	0.18
Peppers, ckd	1.40	0.93	0.59	0.24	tr
Potatoes, raw	0.50	3.51	2.49	1.02	tr
Tomatoes, fresh	0.50	1.40	0.65	0.45	0.30
Tomatoes, cnd	0.40	0.85	0.45	0.37	0.03
Turnips, raw	0.90	2.20	1.50	0.70	tr
Miscellaneous					
Cocoa, concentrate	4.30	43.27	11.25	4.13	27.9
Coffee, instant	tr	16.41	15.55	0.53	0.33
Jam, plum	1.00	0.96	0.80	0.14	0.03
Jam, strawberry	1.00	1.12	0.85	0.11	0.15

TABLE 1. Dietary Fiber (Plantix) Content of Various Foods (Continued)
(g/100 g edible portion)

Food	Crude fiber[1]	Total Dietary fiber (Plantix)[2]	Noncellulosic Polysaccharides[2]	Cellulose[2]	Lignin[2]
Miscellaneous, continued					
Marmalade	1.00	0.71	0.64	0.05	0.01
Pickle	0.50	1.53	0.91	0.50	0.12
Potato chips	1.60	3.20	2.05	1.12	0.03

[1]Department of Agriculture (1). In some cases a crude fiber value could not be found.
In certain instances values are averages.

[2]Adapted from Southgate, et al. (3). Southgate defines dietary fiber as follows:

Dietary fiber =
   Unavailable carbohydrate

Unavailable carbohydrate =
   Noncellulosic polysaccharides +
   Fiber

Noncellulosic polysaccharides =
   Gums +
   Mucilages +
   Algal polysaccharides +
   Pectic substances +
   Hemicelluloses

Fiber =
   Cellulose +
   Lignin (a noncarbohydrate)

TABLE 2.   Certain Dietary Fiber Fractions of Various Foods
(percent dry matter)

Food	Indigestible Residue[1]	Cell wall[2] (NDF)
Grains and grain products		
Soy flour	11.9	--
Bran, bakers	--	37.2
Bran, cereal	--	45.4
Bran, wheat	56.0	--
Oats, rolled	8.2	--
Rice, polished	1.6	--
Bread, rye	21.0	--
Bread, white	4.0	2.4
Bread, whole-wheat	15.5	10.6
Bread, Bran'nola®	--	6.7
Bread, Fresh Horizons®	--	18.4
Bread, Less®	--	16.8
All-Bran®	--	33.9
Cheerios®	--	6.5
Cornflakes	--	4.4
Grape-Nuts®	--	8.2
Heartland®	--	7.4
Porridge oats	--	6.9
Puffed Wheat®	--	7.6
Shredded Wheat®	--	13.4
Wheat Chex®	--	9.6
Wheaties®	--	11.1
Fruits		
Apples	~7	7.6
Oranges, peeled	--	3.7
Pears	~8	--
Legumes (dried) and nuts		
Beans, kidney, ckd	15.0	--
Beans, soy	5.1	--
Beans, white, cnd	15.7	--
Peas, cnd	13.2	--
Peas, dun, cnd	19.6	--
Peanuts, roasted	8.0	--

TABLE 2.   Certain Dietary Fiber Fractions
of Various Foods (Continued)

(percent dry matter)

Food	Indigestible residue[1]	Cell wall[2] (NDF)
Vegetables		
Artichoke hearts	--	12.5
Asparagus	--	12.6
Beans, green	--	17.6
Beans, lima	--	11.9
Beans, wax	--	18.7
Beetroot	--	11.8
Broccoli	--	18.4
Brussel sprouts	~14	21.9
Cabbage	~18	14.2
Cabbage, red	~20	--
Carrots	~13	9.2
Cauliflower	--	16.0
Celery	--	14.4
Collard greens	--	18.6
Corn, kernel	--	7.9
Cucumber, peeled	--	12.7
Cucumber, skin	--	35.5
Eggplant, peeled	--	21.8
Kale	--	16.5
Lettuce, romaine	--	17.3
Mustard greens	--	21.7
Okra	--	14.1
Onions, ckd	~8	7.6
Peas, black-eyed	--	9.0
Peas, green	--	13.3
Pepper, seedless	--	17.2
Potatoes, peeled	--	2.5
Potatoes, skin	9.9	12.9
Radishes	--	14.3
Rutabaga, peeled	--	10.2

TABLE 2.   Certain Dietary Fiber Fractions
of Various Foods (Continued)

(percent dry matter)

Food	Indigestible residue[1]	Cell wall[2] (NDF)
Vegetables, continued		
Spinach	--	17.6
Squash, summer	--	11.4
Squash, zucchini	--	12.5
Turnips, ckd	~20	--
Turnip greens	--	19.4

[1]Values adapted from Hellendoorn et al. (2). Hellendoorn
defines indigestible residue as follows: indigestible
residue = cellulose + hemicellulose + lignin. Pectins,
gums, and mucilages are not included.

[2]By the amylase modification. Values adapted from Robertson
et al. (5). Robertson defines cell wall as follows: cell
wall = lignin + cellulose + hemicellulose. Pectins, gums,
and mucilages are not included.

REFERENCES

1.   Department of Agriculture, Handbook No. 8, Composition
of Foods, Washington, D.C., 1963.

2.   Hellendoorn, E. W., Noordhoff, M. G., and Slagman, J.,
1975, Enzymatic determination of the indigestible residue (dietary fibre) content of human food, J. Sci. Fd.
Agric., 26:1461-1468.

3.   Southgate, D. A. T., Bailey, B., Collinson, E., and
Walker, A., 1976, A guide to calculating intakes of
dietary fibre, J. Human Nutr., 30:303-313.

4.   Spiller, G. A., and Amen, R. J., 1975, Dietary fiber in
human nutrition, CRC Crit. Rev., Food Sci. Nutr., 7:39.

5. Spiller, G. A., and Amen, R. J., <u>Topics</u> <u>in</u> <u>Fiber</u> <u>in</u>
    <u>Human</u> <u>Nutrition</u>, Chapter 1, "The Detergent System of
    Fiber Analysis," by J. B. Robertson, Plenum, 1977,
    in press.

6. Spiller, G. A., Fasset-Cornelius, G., and Briggs, G. M.,
    A new term for plant fibers in nutrition, Am. J. Clin.
    Nutr., <u>29</u>:934.

7. Spiller, G. A., and Shipley, E. A., 1976, New perspec-
    tives on dietary fiber, Food Prod. Dev., <u>10</u>:54-64.

CONTRIBUTORS

Lorne A. Campbell, Ph.D.
Formerly Comparative Pharmacologist
Sunkist Growers, Inc.
Sherman Oaks, California

Anthony J. Gordon, Ph.D.
Former Research Fellow
Department of Animal Physiology
University of Wageningen
The Netherlands

Mervin G.H. Hardinge, M.D., Dr. P.H., Ph.D.
Dean, School of Health
Loma Linda University
Loma Linda, California

Emile W. Hellendoorn, Ph.D.
Central Institute for Nutrition and Food Research TNO
Zeist, The Netherlands

Margaret E. Hendrikx, RD
Chief Metabolic Dietitian
Phoenix Clinical Research Section
National Institute of Arthritis, Metabolism, and
  Digestive Diseases
Phoenix, Arizona

Michael Kliks, M.S.
Research Scientist
Division of Entomology and Parasitology
University of California, Berkeley
Berkeley, California

Grant H. Palmer, B.S.
Research Chemist (retired)
Research Department
Sunkist Growers, Inc.
Ontario, California

James B. Robertson, Ph.D.
Chemical Analyst
Animal Science Department
Cornell University
Ithaca, New York

Robert M. Saunders, Ph.D.
Research Leader
Cereal Products Research Unit
Western Regional Research Laboratory
Agricultural Research Service, U.S. Department
  of Agriculture
Berkeley, California

Elizabeth A. Shipley, B.S., R.D.
Research Nutritionist
Department of Nutritional Science
Syntex Research
Palo Alto, California

SUBJECT INDEX

Acid extraction, 6, 92-93, 105

Acids, 7, 8, 20, 33, 46, 59, 70-72, 80, 84, 86, 91, 105,
    110, 112-113, 150, 151, 152, 156, 160, 161

  in feces, 142, 149, 157, 159, 160

  as products of fermentation, 110, 135, 142-143, 145-146,
    149

Alcohols, 67, 70-71, 86

Alkali, 78, 80, 82, 87, 91

  extraction, 6, 90, 92-93, 105, 128

Bacteria (see Micro-organisms)

Beans

  digestibility of, 137

  extracted, 140, 142, 143, 148

  fiber in, 20, 131, 132, 148, 160, 206, 209

  as gas formers, 137-146

  starch in, 137, 150

  and stool volume, 150

  and transit time, 145-153

Bile, 156, 158, 159, 160

  acid, 155-161, 169, 171, 174

  salt, 60, 155, 157, 160, 169, 171, 174, 175

Bowel (see Colon)

Bran, 22, 117, 120, 121, 128, 132, 154, 170, 171, 172, 173,
    174, 205, 209

  composition of, 47-49, 170

  digestibility of, 49-50, 171-172